# ENOUGH ALREADY

# Enough Already

Learning to Love the
Way I Am Today

VALERIE BERTINELLI

MARINER BOOKS

Boston   New York

marinerbooks.com

Library of Congress Cataloging-in-Publication Data has been applied for.
ISBN 978-0-358-56736-3 (hardcover) | ISBN 978-0-358-62608-4 (signed edition)
ISBN 978-0-358-56732-5 (e-book) | ISBN 978-0-358-62896-5 (audiobook)

Book design by Kelly Dubeau Smydra
All photographs courtesy of the author

1 2021
4500843606

for you ♡

# Contents

# *A Note from Me*

## MAY 2021

ABOUT A YEAR AGO, after an online cooking demonstration, a friend of a friend reached out to me about a difficult situation. At sixty years old, she had finally met a man who, she said, was the love of her life and then he was diagnosed with neck and throat cancer. It had just happened, and they were gearing up to fight it. She asked if I could connect them to my former husband, Edward Van Halen, so they could get the latest and best information on where to go and whom to see for treatment. Ed knew quite a bit about this particular type of cancer from his own long battle with the disease.

I was happy to help.

But something about *my* tone of voice must have hinted at my own troubled state of mind, because at the end of our conversation, in a tone of voice that was slightly softer and more intimate than before, she said, "Hey, if you ever need to talk," and she gave me her number. I thanked her, but I later wondered which of the issues bothering me she had heard in my voice, and I thought, *No way, I'm too private, I don't know her that well, and this stuff I am thinking about is all too personal, anyway.*

Then I caught myself. I went on the *Today* show and sobbed my eyes out. I shared my heart on Instagram. Why was I putting up walls?

Consider the walls down. Let's talk. I have been on a journey with many of you since I was a teenager. I have dated, married, become a mother, divorced, remarried, battled with my weight, and struggled with my self-esteem and mental health. I have also become an empty nester, helped my mother and father through their golden years, and said tearful goodbyes to the people closest to me. I suspect all of you reading this book have gone through many, if not all, of these same issues. I feel like we have done it together as we have grown up.

For you, this book may seem like a new message from me. I see it as a deeper understanding of what I was and still am trying to achieve.

In the past, I have shared my efforts to lose weight and encouraged many of you to do the same. I set certain goals, believing that I would be happier once I lost those ten, twenty, or thirty pounds — or whatever the number was at the time. Then I hit a wall. I was about to begin 2020 resolved to lose ten pounds — the same ten or so pounds I had been trying to lose for more than forty years — and one day, as I embarked on the same morning path from bed to bathroom to scale, I stopped, looked at myself in the mirror, and in a "before coffee" moment of sanity, I said, "No. Stop. I can't be doing this again." And I didn't.

I have come to realize there is no magic number. The scale doesn't light up and set off bells and whistles the way a slot machine does when you hit the jackpot in Las Vegas. The thing I have been looking for can't be quantified. I want to feel true joy inside, and that is very different from wanting to feel thin or see a certain number on the scale.

These days, instead of controlling what I put into myself, I am trying to embrace the many choices I have. My previous books have reflected the mindset of someone who always felt broken. I looked in the mirror and saw flaws and imperfections. I was always trying to fix something about myself. I was always telling myself "No" or "Don't" or "You were bad today" or "You cheated." Why couldn't I see the best of me instead? Why couldn't I see all the good things about myself? Why couldn't I bring myself to say, "Yes!"

This book is about letting go of certain behavior that no longer serves me, recognizing that perhaps it never did, and trying to find new ways of channeling my thoughts and emotions. It's about my efforts to, at sixty-one years old, set aside the landmines of denial, negativity, and self-hate and instead identify values like joy, gratitude, compassion, and forgiveness and try to align with them every day. As I will tell you more than once, these feelings don't find you. You have to go in search of them, knowing some days will be better than others, none will be perfect, but that is life.

And this book is about grief—a topic I didn't intend to write about and hoped not to, and yet it was unavoidable. Any search for joy has to include the reverse side of the picture, and that is grief. The two are partners in this dance of ours.

To write this book, I looked inside myself the way I do the fridge when I have an idea for a new take on a favorite recipe and I began to pull out ingredients. They weren't necessarily all the ingredients that I intended or thought I was going to use, so when everything was on the counter, my original idea took on a momentum of its own. It became a collection of thoughts, essays, and stories—roughly chronological but connected by the frazzled threads of my life—that eventually, after much pulling and tugging at my heart, made sense to me.

My hope is that they make sense to you, too. I wrote about the things that I have gone through and continue to deal with as I got to where I am today at age sixty-one, topics that I think will be familiar to many of you—being a mom, making midlife career changes, caring for aging parents, asking why the hell have I been so hard on myself for so long, saying goodbye to those I love, recognizing mistakes, and searching for meaning. Anything sound familiar?

I endeavored to share my experiences and thoughts about growing older with the emphasis on the effort to grow. I believe we are here to learn lessons. It's not all sunny days and roses. But there is enough warmth and perfume to remind us that life is a gift—and too short to waste.

You are going to find me frequently using the words "me" and "I" in this book. They appear far too often for my taste, but, hey, my name is on the book. What I would like you to do, though, is substitute yourself in various places. Where it says "me" or "I," think of how these stories are like your own. Our lives may be different, but I sense that the situations we face and the questions we ask ourselves are very similar.

I draw strength from knowing so many of you are out there supporting me. You should know that I am there for you, too. I really hope this book provides you with the comfort I have found while writing it. Hug the people you love. And hug yourself. (Don't put it off. Do it today. Right now. I'll wait.)

This is a love story. I've tried to share experiences that have taught me about hope, joy, happiness, forgiveness, kindness, and love. Most of all love. As I move forward in life, I continue to learn it's only and all about love in the end.

Valerie

Studio City, California

# Learning to Love the Way I Am

## *My (Try) To-Do List*

### SEPTEMBER 2019

1. Drink a lot of water
2. Eat a big breakfast, an average lunch, and a tiny dinner
3. Eat more vegetables and fruits
4. Avoid processed food
5. Go for a walk, swim, or bike ride
6. Don't forget to stretch
7. Read a book
8. Go to bed earlier
9. STOP thinking negative thoughts about yourself and other people
10. Don't judge or compare yourself to others
11. Enjoy the little things in life
12. Begin yoga or meditation
13. STOP procrastinating — do not put things off
14. Live in the moment
15. Don't dwell on the past
16. Listen to peaceful music

17. Live in a tidy place
18. Wear clothes that make you happy
19. Donate or throw away things you don't need
20. Breathe
21. Exhale
22. GO OUTSIDE
23. GO OUTSIDE THE NEXT DAY AND THE NEXT . . .
24. Remember that the effort you make will be rewarded

# Before You Begin, a Suggestion

Before you read any further, may I suggest making this snack and finding a comfortable place to sit down and enjoy the first chapter. You will understand why soon enough.

## Hot Spinach and Crab Dip

2   tablespoons unsalted butter

1   small onion, finely chopped

1   clove garlic, finely chopped

    Kosher salt

    Freshly ground black pepper

8   ounces cream cheese

1   teaspoon Worcestershire sauce

½   teaspoon dry mustard

½   teaspoon paprika

⅛   teaspoon cayenne pepper

1   pound frozen chopped spinach, thawed and squeezed very dry

8   ounces lump crabmeat, picked through for bits of shell

½   cup shredded Monterey Jack

3   tablespoons grated Parmesan

2   tablespoons panko bread crumbs

    Crackers, for serving

*(recipe continued on next page)*

Preheat the oven to 425 degrees F.

Melt the butter in a medium pot over medium heat.

Add the onion and garlic, season with salt and pepper to taste, and cook, stirring occasionally, until softened, about 6 minutes.

Add the cream cheese, Worcestershire sauce, dry mustard, paprika, and cayenne pepper, and stir until melted.

Add the spinach and crabmeat, and stir until warm and bubbling. Stir in the Monterey Jack and Parmesan, and season with salt and pepper.

Transfer the dip to a small baking dish and top with the panko bread crumbs. Place the baking dish on a baking sheet and bake until bubbling and golden, about 15 minutes.

Serve hot with crackers.

# The Clock Is Ticking

## OCTOBER 2019

**P**URE FUN. THAT IS what I am experiencing when I make a cheesy spinach and crab dip on *The Kelly Clarkson Show*. I am glammed up for TV and leading Kelly and actress-singer Hailee Steinfeld through the easy-to-follow and oh-so-yummy steps of this dish. We also get a little dishy, and I tell the story of how I was once mistaken for Kelly's mom when I was in the audience of *American Idol*, and Kelly asks me about the correct pronunciation of Worcestershire sauce, explaining that she likes it in her Bloody Marys.

Suddenly, the two of us pretend to slur our words. We get very silly; though as we do, a little voice in my head reminds me to keep one eye on the dip and never stop stirring. That might be the secret to success in everything, right? *Keep one eye on the dip and never stop stirring.* Interpret as you wish.

With onions and garlic simmering in a pot, I add a block of cream cheese, cayenne pepper, paprika, mustard, pepper, some fresh crabmeat, spinach, Monterey Jack, Parmesan, and a sprinkle of panko bread crumbs. Once the ingredients are mixed together and warm, I transfer them to another dish that gets popped into the oven for about fifteen minutes. The finished dish gets raves from Kelly, Hailee, and the crew.

I leave the studio with leftovers, and the next day I take them to my son's house. I also bring some crackers and crudités. What twenty-eight-year-old guy keeps cut-up raw vegetables on hand? I also have an ulterior motive. It is October 2019, and Wolfie has been working on his first album, which does not yet have a release date, but he does have more than a dozen songs and I want him to put all of them on my phone so I can listen to them whenever I want, which will be practically all the time.

Yes, I am a proud mom—and for good reason. He has written all the songs and played all the instruments. I think the songs are amazing. I want the dip to buy me enough time to listen, get him to help me with the download, and ask all sorts of mom questions. When we inevitably get to the point where he has had enough of my prying, I will say, "How about that dip?"

The plan works. At Wolfie's, I head straight to the kitchen as I usually do when I visit him. I often bring groceries or a meal to heat up. This time it is the cheesy spinach and crab dip. He has a sleek, modern kitchen that opens up to a living room and dining room. It feels like a bright, airy loft. I turn on the oven and heat up the dip. I wipe my hands on a dish towel that I half remember buying him a while ago and ask Wolfie what is new. He catches me up on this and that, then he casually says, "By the way, Dad is on his way over."

"Dad" is my ex-husband and friend, Edward Van Halen—Ed to me.

"That's great," I say. "I haven't seen him in a while. How's he feeling?"

"He's okay," Wolfie says.

Wolfie explains that Ed had called while I was on my way over to his house. He was out doing errands with his assistant and asked if he could drop by for a visit. A few minutes later, as I am setting the warm dip on the kitchen counter, Ed knocks and opens the door. He stops a couple of steps inside after hearing Wolfie's music playing on the sound system. His face turns into one big smile. "How about this kid?" he says to me as we hug. "I know," I say. "My heart is melting."

So is the spinach and crab dip. But Ed spots the bowl on the kitchen counter and suddenly this impromptu meeting of the two copresidents of the Wolfgang Van Halen Fan Club is paused. He walks over to the dish and smells it.

"What'd you make?" he asks.

As I answer, he pops a cracker with a giant scoop of dip into his mouth.

"Wow."

He dives in for seconds and thirds, standing over the dip, elbows on each side of the bowl, as if he has taken it hostage. He doesn't realize that he is hogging it for himself.

"Dad, it's for everybody," Wolfie says, smiling.

Ed laughs and steps back with another cracker full of dip in his hand. "Oh, sorry. But, Val, this is amazing."

Ed and I stopped living together in 2002 and divorced in 2007. Both of us remarried, but in our own way, we stayed together. We have shared four decades of love, anger, frustration, friendship, and love. That is what has endured—the love. And that is the lesson I have learned and continue to learn, especially these days.

The same is true for Ed, who was diagnosed with tongue cancer in 2000 and has been battling different forms of the damn disease ever since. He has been having a particularly rough go of it lately. That is what makes seeing him eat with such relish a particularly joyous occasion. At sixty-four years old, he is still devilishly cute. But at this moment, what matters even more is that he still seems to like my cooking.

. . . . . . . . .

I first met Ed backstage at a Van Halen concert in Shreveport, Louisiana. My brother knew someone who got us VIP passes. Ed was shy. We said hello before the show and talked for a long time afterward until it was time for the band to get on their bus. The attraction was instantaneous and mutual. Some people observed that we looked remarkably alike, like brother and sister. Our connection was deep right from the start.

A short time later, I met him on the road when the band was still on tour, and I was even more smitten. He was adorable, introverted, and possessed by a vulnerability as prodigious as his talent.

For me, it was almost incidental that this twenty-five-year-old was already considered the greatest rock guitarist of his generation. It seemed overwhelming to him, though. At the time, Ed and his brother, Alex, still lived with their parents in Pasadena. They were too busy chasing rock stardom to get a place of their own. They weren't home that much anyway, probably because when they were, they had to deal with their taskmaster mother.

Mrs. Van Halen was a tough, demanding woman who wasn't easy on her boys, rock stars or not—and, in fact, she didn't approve of the lifestyle of a touring musician. But whatever issues they had were set aside when she put food on the table. Ed and Alex loved her cooking. She made all of their favorite Indonesian dishes—sambal chicken, *gado-gado, spekkoek,* and *pisang goreng*—and the beasts were temporarily tamed.

Food was something Ed and I responded to differently. Although he could enjoy a home-cooked meal, more often than not, he ate only because he got hungry and knew he had to eat to keep going. I ate because I loved food, and later on, I used food as a substitute for love. It was one of the reasons I took notice of the way Ed sat over the spinach and crab dip. He loved the way it tasted. I wanted to believe he was savoring much more.

When Ed's father learned we were dating, he told his son that I was only a teenager and way too young for him. Ed explained to his father that he was watching reruns of my TV series, *One Day at a Time*. In reality, I was two weeks shy of twenty-one years old when we got married and totally legal and perfectly in love. Ed felt the same way. We were portrayed as a mismatch: a bad-boy rock star and America's sweetheart. It made for juicy reading. But privately, Ed wasn't the person people thought he was and neither was I. He was shy, and I was loud. We got along very well when he wasn't drinking or using drugs, and I'm convinced we would have stayed together if not for some crazy, cliché eighties-style behavior.

Our split was hard and complicated by the fact that we had a child who both of us agreed was our best creation. While we often lived very different lives in the ten years after Wolfie was born, we never lived them separately. Wolfie kept us together and, more important, ensured that we remained a tightly bonded threesome. After we split, an ironic thing happened. Ed and I grew even closer together. We couldn't live with each other, but we found it impossible to live completely apart. I won't say we wrote our own happy ending. It was more like To Be Continued . . .

· · · · · · · · ·

*So Ed looks good*, I think, after a careful and what I hope is an inconspicuous but thorough assessment. He's wearing a red knit shirt and khakis, and with his hair short, he resembles a golf pro more than he does a rock god, and I think that he would be thrilled with a superstar golf game at this point in time.

I sit down next to him and am inclined to put my arm around him and give him a friendly, affectionate squeeze, but as is often typical of me, I overthink this simple, natural, innocent gesture and sit there with my hands in my lap. I don't want to appear inappropriate, do something that might be misinterpreted, or intrude on his space, though when Ed arrived, he gave me a kiss and a hug, and asked, "How ya doing?"

It was so easy and natural for him.

How come I am so weird and uptight?

I am sure it has something to do with my awareness that his second marriage is basically over, as he confided a while ago, and also with the fact that my own second marriage is in trouble, which I haven't told anyone. They are two unrelated situations, and there is no chance we are going to get back together. But I do know if one of us were to open up, the other would too, and I don't want to get into that. Not here. Not now.

I simply wish I was more comfortable letting him know how much I love him. The spinach and crab dip will have to suffice for now.

A year later, I will think how stupid that was. I should have just put my arm around him. I should have. Ugh. "Should have" is a terrible place to live.

Accidental get-togethers like this are more common than not for us. Other than Wolfie's birthday, though, we don't plan family time as much as we rely on it to just happen. I don't think either of us were ever good planners and we haven't improved over time. We also have our separate lives. It just happens that those separate lives frequently intersect. I think the last time I saw Ed was at one of Wolfie's band rehearsals four or five months ago when both of us showed up without knowing the other one was going to be there.

That was emotional. I could close my eyes and picture myself on the side of the stage at a Van Halen concert and watching Ed play with the biggest grin on his face. The only time I saw his famous smile get bigger was when he watched Wolfie play. He poured all the pride he never let himself feel about his own ability into Wolfie. I loved hearing him say, "You're a beast. You're amazing." He meant it.

In 2006, when Wolfie was only fifteen, he began jamming with Ed and his uncle Alex in 5150, Ed's backyard studio. A year later, Ed brought him into the family business. It was a helluva way for both of them to grow up; for me, it was a fast track to more gray hair and meant giving up the control I was used to as his mom. More recently, the two of them were spending nearly every day together. Wolfie was driving his dad to all of his doctor appointments, and when Ed was in the hospital, Wolfie visited him two or three times a day. And sometimes even spent the night.

I was so proud of the young man Wolfie had become. It was so fun to lean into Ed, and say, "Look what we did. Pretty good, eh?"

This kid, who was not a kid anymore except to the two of us, was the thing Ed and I got right. He was the best of both of us. He worked extremely hard not only to learn Van Halen's songs but to perfect them, because that's the only level his father would accept, and he did it playing bass, an instrument that was fairly new to him. From the moment I got pregnant, Ed dreamed of playing with the baby growing inside me. Girl or boy, it didn't matter to him. He wanted to play music with this child. And he did. They played together on three world tours and two Van Halen albums. Ed was in heaven; I had never seen him smile so much. He was playing alongside his brother and his son.

Ed also taught Wolfie to ignore the naysayers and critics or give them the middle finger if he ran out of tolerance. I admired my son for never losing his ability to laugh off most things and shrug off the worst. He had more patience than either his dad or I had.

Starting in 2015, Wolfie began recording his own music. However, before he ever recorded a single note, he spent years practicing and writing. He explored the music inside him and brought it to the surface, sometimes with ease and other times it came out kicking and screaming. Even when your first and last names are synonymous with music, art is not easy to make, and in fact, having names that echo greatness may make it harder to create.

Ed and I were never happier than when we saw Wolfie dig deep into himself and the joy he got from playing us something he had made. I was transported back to the days when I volunteered in his elementary school classroom. He always wanted to show me his work, grinning as he said, "Look, Ma," and eagerly waiting to get a hug. Wolfie's dad saw and heard something more in his solo effort. To Ed, it was his own past and his son's future. It was the passing of the torch, something he had started when he gave Wolfie a drum kit for his tenth birthday, then brought him onstage at Van Halen's 2004 concerts for alternating guitar solos on "316," a song that Ed had written years before and played softly on my belly all through my pregnancy. When Wolfie was born on March 16, it became his song.

Wolfie finished his solo album in 2018 and formed a band, intending to go out on tour. But his plans were put on hold after we got the news that Ed's cancer had spread and turned into stage IV lung cancer. This was the latest chapter in an ongoing story, but it was an ominous turn of events that made both Ed and Wolfie acutely aware that the clock was ticking. Most of us don't bother to pay attention. Once you hear the ticktock of mortality, you can't unhear it. It's not a bad thing. Neither does it have to be a depressing thing. It's a reminder.

· · · · · · · · ·

All of us are mortal. Our lives have a beginning, a middle, and an end. It's something that seems to happen without much consideration outside of life's biggest and unavoidable moments: graduations, marriages, breakups, birthdays, and deaths. For most of us, life is a gradual climb up a ladder. It's punctuated by different milestones, like turning forty, fifty, sixty, and so on. Our children grow up and move out and establish independent lives of their own. We become empty nesters and reevaluate our lives. We find ourselves taking care of our parents and, at some point, tearfully saying goodbye to them.

I knew this firsthand. I had experienced all of the above.

Inevitably, though, the ladder we're climbing will wobble. Nothing bad might happen, but later it moves again, this time a little harder—or maybe a lot harder, hard enough that you lose your balance. For Ed, the wobble happened when he was first diagnosed with cancer. Then it got to where he was holding on so he wouldn't fall off.

At that point, he knew the most precious thing he had and the only thing that mattered was time. Wolfie, though only in his mid-twenties, knew that, too.

I have the uncanny ability to not think about such things until I have no choice, then I can't not think about them. It's the reason both Wolfie and Ed keep some of the details about Ed's illness from me. They don't want me to worry more than I already do. So, although I don't know the extent of Ed's illness, I know it's serious, and seeing the way he scarfs down my spinach and crab dip, I want to do something nice for him.

"You should come over and I'll make you *bami*," I say.

Bami is basically an Indonesian-Dutch stir-fry with noodles, pork, and veggies. There are multiple ways to spell it—*bahmi*, *bakmi*, and *bami goreng*—and even more recipes than spellings. I bet every Indonesian woman has her own variation. I got mine from Ed's mom. After Ed and I got married, he went on the road to tour the band's latest album and I stayed in LA. I had my work and career. I stayed with Ed's parents as a way to get to know my in-laws. They lived in a house that Ed and Alex had bought them.

Ed's mom was a tiny, acerbic, outspoken Indonesian woman with very set ways that all boiled down to her way. She spent the boys' childhood trying to exert control, and I sensed that she regularly came out on the losing end of that tug-of-war. Though the boys respected her, they still did what they wanted. Now that they were grown up, she ran the house her way. She was a pack rat. She went to Costco and Kmart a couple of times a week and came back with more of everything. I was amused the first time I saw this, because it was only she and Ed's dad in the house, yet the shelves were stocked with rows and rows of canned goods, paper towels, and toilet paper. She could've opened her own store.

Or restaurant. When she cooked for Ed and me, she usually made *gado-gado*, a vegetable salad with hard-boiled eggs and a peanut dipping sauce; or a spicy chicken dish that I never got the recipe for and am still trying to perfect; or her bami. She might have had recipes lying around somewhere, maybe tucked in a drawer, but I doubt it. She just knew what to do. It's the place where I have finally arrived when I make my Bolognese.

While I was staying with her and Pa—we called Ed's parents Ma and Pa—I began to marvel at the coffee she made in the morning. I only call it coffee because that's what I saw her spoon into her French press, along with cream and sugar. The result was the most delicious cup of coffee I had ever had. I have tried countless times to replicate it and have never succeeded, which is why I have my reservations about calling it coffee.

Whatever it was, I relished that morning brew, which she served with a piece of buttered toast and a paper-thin slice of ham and cheese (I think it was a hard white cheddar). I have no idea what magical way she buttered that toast and layered the other ingredients, but it was perfection. I would let that first bite linger on the top of my tongue in order to enjoy the mix of sweet and savory as if it were the good-morning hug I was missing from Ed. I asked Ma to teach me how to make these things, not the morning toast and coffee, but Ed's favorites, her Indonesian specialties. She graciously agreed.

We started with bami. But I quickly realized that her method of instruction was the same as my grandmother's when she showed me how she made gnocchi. It turns out that there is no difference between little old Indonesian women and little old Italian women. Mrs. Van Halen essentially told me to do a little of this and a little of that, and when I looked up at her with uncertainty about the next steps, she patted me on the back, and said, "You can do it." I might as well have been a six-year-old going off the high dive for the first time.

Watching her make *ketjap sambal,* the sauce for the bami, was akin to watching Derek DelGaudio do a card trick. She magically mixed some soy sauce and brown sugar, then added a diced pepper into the simmering sauce as if she were sprinkling fairy dust over it. Once, we made *spekkoek* together. *Spekkoek* is described as an Indonesian-Dutch layer cake consisting of multiple thin layers of cake with alternating flavors like cinnamon and vanilla that are all drenched in butter. The list of ingredients includes egg yolks, butter, sugar, nutmeg, cardamom, ginger, cloves, and more butter. Every layer needed to be made individually, it took all day, and it was heavenly.

· · · · · · · · ·

Before leaving Wolfie's, I invite Ed to dinner the next day. "I want to make you bami," I tell him. He responds with a grin that lights up his face.

"Bami, oh my God," he says. "I haven't had that in forever. You'd make that for me?"

"Of course, I'll make it for you," I say. "Do you want it with pork or turkey?"

"Pork," he says.

"Do you remember the last time I made bami with your mom?" I ask. "It was Thanksgiving when I was pregnant with Wolfie. She came over to help me, and after a few minutes, she ended up shoving me to the side and making it herself."

We laugh.

"It was delicious," I say.

Later, before saying goodbye, I mention again that I am looking forward to making him dinner. It's like I want to take both of us back to a different time. Past invitations have been cancelled for one reason or another. But this time I sense that I no longer have that kind of luxury, and I think Ed feels the same way.

Unfortunately, Ed calls a couple of hours before dinner and cancels. He says that he isn't feeling well and that he hopes I understand.

I assure him that I do understand and offer a rain check. Then I hang up the phone and cry.

· · · · · · · · ·

The next time I see Ed is at Thanksgiving. I can't remember the last time he joined the usual roundup of family and close friends for this annual November feast, but he gladly accepted the invi-

tation and was chauffeured over by his friend and golfing buddy
George Lopez. The two of them are unlikely besties who bonded
years earlier over their mutually masochistic enjoyment of playing
eighteen holes of golf. Ed's caregiver, Leon, is also with them.

When they arrive, the house is bustling with people, including
Wolfie and his longtime girlfriend, Andraia; my brother Patrick
and his wife, Stacy; and several others, including Matt Bruck, Ed's
longtime right-hand man, and Matt's mother.

Most of us are standing around the kitchen island talking and
catching up, with the major topic of inquiry being Wolfie's progress on his debut album. Some people make brief sorties into out-
lying rooms to get snacks and check on the scores of various football games. A TV is set up in nearly every room, a tribute to my
obsession with football.

Back when I was working on *Hot in Cleveland,* Wendie Malick
once said, "Before we met, I had this impression of you as a sweet,
timid little thing. But you're actually quite the truck driver." I can't
deny it. I am kind of a bull in a china shop.

I am also a diehard New Orleans Saints fan, and they are in
one of three NFL games being played Thanksgiving Day, so I am
among those who slip in and out of the room for updates.

It's on one of these trips that I run into Ed as he walks through
the front door. I give him a hug and a kiss, and note that he looks
good, no different than he had a few weeks earlier and maybe even
a little better. I see a brightness in his eyes that conveys his happiness at being with us at the house. I am really glad that he has
come, that he is feeling well enough, and that he is able to partic-
ipate in the rituals of being together as a family—acknowledging
our connections, re-establishing our ties to each other, debating,
reminiscing, laughing, and eating as much as we can possibly hold.

Ed is already smiling and nodding at people as I encourage him
to settle in and remind him that I have made bami for him. He in-

hales deeply, savoring the various aromas wafting from the kitchen, and says that it smells delicious.

"I hope so," I say.

· · · · · · · · ·

The meal has not been without last-minute concerns. The pumpkin pie—Wolfie's favorite—which I made the night before, didn't turn out because I mistakenly used sweetened condensed milk instead of evaporated milk as called for in the recipe. When I cut a slice and tasted it early in the morning, it was way too sweet and just godawful.

In the morning, I make an emergency run to the grocery store and buy ingredients to make a whole new pumpkin pie, including a store-bought pie crust (no judgment, please—I am trying to save time). Back home, I am a blur of activity. I make the pie, get it in the oven, and start on the ketjap for the bami. Knowing the pie bakes for an hour, I set the timer, put the ketjap on simmer, and run upstairs to shower.

When I come back down, my heart sinks a little. The pie smells amazing, but I can smell the ketjap burning. I react by screaming a few choice words. Wolfie and my brother come into the kitchen to see what has happened, and I snap, "Couldn't one of you have turned off the flame under the ketjap?"

They shrug.

"Oh, that's what that smell was." Patrick laughs.

"Yes, that's what that smell was," I say.

"Sorry. Guess you burned it."

It's lucky that I have enough ingredients to make another batch of ketjap. And this time I keep an eye on the simmer.

Such is Valerie's home cooking, Thanksgiving edition.

· · · · · · · · ·

By the time we sit down at the table, everything is on track. I kick off the feast with a toast to family, the blessing of food and health, and my beloved Saints, who are in the process of serving the Falcons some Thanksgiving whoop-ass. The noise level swells as we rip into the meal. Everyone eats with a gusto reflective of people who have waited a year for this favorite meal. The turkey, which started off at twenty-six pounds, disappears off the platter. The mashed potatoes are a hit, too. I love the stuffing, and Ed is happy with just the bami.

Every time I glance at him, he is nibbling a little bit more. This is the magic of food and the reason I delight in preparing it. In the right context, like this one, food is more than a meal. It is a joyous ride back to tables of the past. One bite opens the door to a chorus of memories from childhood and family and special occasions. It is comfort and love.

Not all of our family holidays have been like this. At one New Year's Eve dinner at our beach house, my dad punched Ed. My then-husband, having imbibed a prodigious amount of Jägermeister, wanted to go for a drive. He was clearly not fit to get behind the wheel. But Ed ignored my stern objections, insisting that he wanted to cruise up and down the coast, and he rather gruffly pushed past me.

My dad stepped in front of Ed, said a few words with paternalistic authority, and attempted to take the keys from his hand. When Ed resisted, my dad punched him. The force of the blow cracked Ed's cheekbone. When Ed blew his nose, his entire cheek puffed up. Joyriding on Pacific Coast Highway was no longer an option. I had to take him to the emergency room.

After forty years together, we have learned to appreciate the good times and laugh through the more difficult moments. Both of us have remarried—Ed in 2009, and me two years later—yet one thing never changed. Every time we saw each other, we made it a point to say I love you. Now more so than ever.

I figure that this is what Ed wants to tell me when he pulls me aside after dessert, and says, "Hey, can I talk to you privately?"

Dishes are being cleared. People have spread out, literally, on sofas and chairs. They stare at the ESPN wrap-up show and talk about how full they are.

"Sure," I say to Ed, looking around for a place where we can have privacy.

Every room is full, so we go outside and get into George Lopez's car. Ed sits in the driver's seat. I slide in the passenger's side, eager to get out of the chilly night air. A few minutes later, after warming up, Ed hands me a small bag and tells me to open it. It's light. I open the smooth black box; inside is a small pendant-size bar of pure gold. I have never seen anything like this. It is mostly plain, but it has a small design on it that I assume was made by a mold. There's beauty in its simplicity and purity.

With tears in his eyes, Ed explains that he bought it the previous year when he was in Germany, where he went to get experimental cancer treatments to stop or slow the spread of his disease. He was collecting gold coins at the time, and this bar had caught his eye and made him think of me.

"I hope you don't think it's weird," he says. "You know, that I bought my ex-wife this gift and I didn't get my wife anything. I just love you."

I shake my head, knowing what he means and sharing that sentiment.

"I love you, too," I say, with tears in my eyes.

Ed reiterates that he was thinking of me, not his wife, Janie, when he was in Germany, and it confused him and made him feel guilty, which he wants to talk about, though, as I suspect, what he really wants to talk about goes much deeper, because how can you not want to go deeper and cut right to the core of what really matters when cancer is ravaging your body and destroying your sense of tomorrow?

For nearly an hour, we sit in the car, inches apart, and open our hearts to each other, sharing our feelings about each other from the start of our relationship to the present. He wants me to know that he messed up and that it is too bad. I agree but acknowledge that I contributed to our troubles, too, and that I am also sorry. It seems odd to be having this conversation now, but I have a simultaneous sense of why not now. And if not now, we may run out of other nows. We waited long enough to get to this point, which is this: the only thing that matters is love, and the two of us love each other.

Crying, Ed goes on to talk about his current relationship, his fears about the progression of his illness, an upcoming back operation, and eventually his appreciation of the bami I made and all the memories it brought back. I realize how much he needed to get all this information and emotion out of him, and how important it is to me, too. I keep my eyes locked on his. I want him to know that I am there for him, always. He is looking for inner peace. He is very brave. He is also scared. And he is just so very, very vulnerable and human.

I don't remember when or how we stop crying, but we do. So many times like this one I have worried that the pain and the tears won't ever end, but they do, and I never remember how or when they did, only that I felt better afterward for having allowed myself to face that situation. Ed seems to feel the same way. We have forgiven each other for the mistakes we made and the pain we caused each other over the past forty years. It's a relief—and freeing. Nothing is left between us but love—and Ed's smile.

A moment or two of quiet follows as we sit there. I feel a deep and profound sense of peace between us. It makes me think of a photograph I have inside the house—which is actually three photos framed together; there's one each of Ed, Wolfie, and me when we all were two years old. The three of us look exactly the same. And I'm the one with the shortest hair.

Ed might be having a similar thought because, before getting out of the car, he says, "Boy, we did make a great son, didn't we?"

I take his hand and hold it tightly in mine. "We did," I say. "We sure did."

· · · · · · · · ·

I am drained and a little disoriented when we walk back inside. Ed doesn't stay much longer. I pour myself a generous glass of white wine and let the night wind down, saying goodbye to people with hugs that are a little tighter and stronger, and appreciating the coziness of my home.

Leftovers are packaged up and put away in the fridge or given to others to take home. The dishwasher is already humming away. I rinse the overflow of dirty dishes and let them sit on the counter; I will deal with them in the morning.

I wish I could be like this more often: sitting with myself and accepting what is, even if it's messy, instead of trying to solve every problem completely or numbing myself with food when I can't or feel overwhelmed.

I am exhausted, but it's a good tired.

I got through it.

*This is the real dessert of Thanksgiving.* Maybe dessert is the wrong idea. Maybe it's the gravy on top of the whole experience.

The walk upstairs to the bedroom is the last mile of a daylong hike. As I get into bed, I notice several books about forgiveness in the stack on my nightstand. How to forgive. Learning how to forgive. The blessing of forgiveness. The lessons in all of them lead to the same place, and I realize that it is surprisingly easy to forgive someone when you love them.

. . . . . . . . .

At the end of December, I spend a few days with Wolfie and Andraia at our old house in Park City, Utah. Wolfie and I have talked about this trip for several years. Ed and I bought this old 1890s mining shack when Wolfie was a preschooler and we sold it about ten years later. We always harbored some regret about doing this. In early 2019, Wolfie found the house listed on Airbnb, which he immediately showed me, and said, "I really want all of us to go there again. You, me, Dad, and all of our friends. People can come and go. It will be like old times."

I loved the idea. We all did. As a result, I did something that I never do: I planned ahead and booked the house over Christmas and New Year's.

When it is time to fly to Park City, Wolfie tries to back out. Ed has to have surgery and Wolfie wants to be there with him. I tell him that Ed's caregiver will be with him and that Park City is only an hour's flight from LA should he need to go back, and that, as his mother, I am concerned about him. I can see he needs some time away to relax.

I am right, too. As soon as we are in the house, I notice Wolfie's shoulders relax and hear him breathe easier. He laughs and jokes more. He makes fun of the pleasure I am having being back here. I can't help it—and don't want to. I can feel our past in the air. Even though the house appears to have been redone more than once since we were last here, it's like we hung our memories in the closet when we left, and they are still there.

When we lived here, the tiny house had an open floor plan and a prominent quirk: the floor sloped. The whole house was on a slight tilt. Wolfie was able to push one of his Matchbox cars from his bedroom and watch it roll all the way to the front door. I hear him telling Andraia about it as well as some other stories of the times we spent here. He was a little boy then and only thirteen when we sold the house, but I can hear him recalling so many details with such color and humor that I can't help but smile. Apparently, we did a few things right as parents.

He and Andraia want to go for a walk into town. I follow them outside and stand on the front porch, watching them walk down the street. I breath in the fresh mountain air; I love it. This house always had a happy vibe, and I am glad to see it's still present. Later that night, we FaceTime with Ed and let him know how much we wish he could be with us.

"Me, too," he says. "When this is over and I'm feeling stronger, maybe we can all go back."

"Definitely," I say.

"Love you, Pop," Wolfie says.

Strange how we have come here to recapture a sense of family, and despite Ed's not being able to make it, we somehow still succeed. He's here with us, on FaceTime and in spirit. I stay for only a few days; Wolfie and Andraia are staying through New Year's. Except for taking a few walks, I don't feel much like going out. Cooking for them is my way of relaxing and spending time with them. I make turkey meatball soup and chicken Marbella. Tonight's dish is shrimp scampi and zoodles, which is Andraia's favorite.

The slow, methodical prep relaxes me; it feels almost like a meditation. As the ingredients simmer, the thick, appealing aroma of garlic and butter fills the house. This is the smell of love meeting divinity. It is all the proof I need to know that God not only exists but wears an apron and, at least in my case, is likely Italian.

The light begins to wane and soon it will drop behind the mountains. The air is crisp and fresh. I am one of those people who seems to end up visiting my old homes on Google when I am looking for something in my life, and here I am. Park City was always special to me. I missed the house, and I missed the love I put into that house. I missed how I felt in that house but coming back is giving me a taste of that again.

Wolfie and Andraia get back from their walk. I hear them laughing before they come inside. Their cheeks are red from the cold. *That's a picture worth remembering*, I tell myself. I am a happy mom. Wolfie tells me that the walk was great and that dinner smells incredible. Then he pulls out his cell phone and holds it up for me to see. He says that he got a text from his dad.

"Oh, what did he say?" I ask.

"He said, 'You're awesome, and I love you.'"

# Bami Goreng

Mrs. Van Halen wasn't always patient with me when she was teaching me how to make this and other favorites. It was like being in the kitchen with an Indonesian Julia Child. Before Thanksgiving, when I was pregnant with Wolfie, I wanted to make this and asked her to help me. She came over to our house, and after a few minutes of watching me try to prepare this dish, she shoved me aside, and said, "Let me do it." She did, and we loved it. Now you try it. I promise I won't shove you aside. Whatever you do, it will be delicious.

### Ketjap Sambal

1 tablespoon canola oil

2 teaspoons minced garlic (1 to 2 cloves)

2 teaspoons grated fresh ginger (a 1-inch knob)

2 teaspoons minced seeded jalapeño

¼ cup packed light brown sugar

¼ cup tamari

½ teaspoon five-spice powder

### Bami Goreng

1 tablespoon canola oil

1 cup thinly sliced red onion (½ onion)

2 teaspoons minced garlic (1 to 2 cloves)

2 teaspoons grated fresh ginger (a 1-inch knob)

1   cup thinly sliced red bell pepper (1 bell pepper)

8   ounces pork tenderloin, sliced into ¼-inch rounds and halved crosswise

Kosher salt

2   cups thinly sliced Napa cabbage

1   tablespoon sambal oelek

8   ounces thin spaghetti, cooked

Lime wedges, for juicing and serving

Roughly chopped cilantro leaves, for garnish

*Make the Ketjap Sambal*

Heat the canola oil in a small saucepot over medium heat.

Stir in the garlic, ginger, and jalapeño, and sauté until fragrant but not yet browned, 2 to 3 minutes. Add the brown sugar, tamari, five-spice powder, and ¼ cup water.

Bring the mixture to a simmer and cook until the sauce reduces and is thick enough to coat the back of a spoon, about 10 minutes. Remove from the heat and set aside.

*Bami Goreng*

Heat the canola oil in a 12-inch sauté pan over high heat.

Add the red onion, garlic, and ginger, and cook until softened.

*(recipe continued on next page)*

Add the red pepper. Sprinkle the pork tenderloin with salt and add it to the pan; cook until browned on both sides, 3 to 4 minutes total.

Add the cabbage, stir in the sambal oelek, then deglaze the pan with ¼ cup water. Cook 2 for 3 minutes until the water is evaporated.

Finally, add in the cooked spaghetti and half of the ketjap sambal.

Transfer the bami goreng to a large bowl and drizzle with the remaining ketjap. Add a squeeze of lime and garnish with cilantro. Serve with extra lime wedges on the side.

**Serves** 4 to 6 people

# Enough Already

## DECEMBER 2019

BACK IN LA, I am thinking about Dexter, the regal Burmese cat who once patrolled our house as if he owned the place. I miss talking to him.

I bought Dexter at a pet store in 2000 (I know, I know, it was the last time I ever did that; I got my next six cats and dog at a shelter) and spent nearly every day with him until cancer cut short his life in 2013. He was a stunning young man. To this day, the screen saver on my phone is a picture of Dexter that Wolfie took in 2006. Dexter liked to nuzzle and be held. He was vocal and always let me know when he was in the room, and he responded in kind—and with kindness—when I needed attention from him. He was my traveling companion, my shadow. He went through the hardest times of my life with me, and I talked to him about everything. A lot of our conversation was my asking, "Oh Dexter, what should I do?" or "What does it mean?"

I wish he were with me now.

The new year is weighing on me. I am scheduled to do a cooking segment on the *Today* show in early January. The show pitched me on becoming a more permanent part of the *Today* family without having to move to New York. I loved the idea. Being around Hoda Kotb, Savannah Guthrie, Al Roker, Natalie Morales, Carson Daly, and the rest of the on-air talent and their producers makes me feel smarter and better informed.

For my first segment, I am going to show how to make a simple, healthy meal and talk about my number one resolution for the new year: losing ten pounds. The production staff has done research and found that losing weight and eating healthier are among the most popular resolutions people make every year. I am one of those people. Every year I resolve to lose ten pounds, exercise more, eat healthier, and blah-blah-blah.

This must be part of the reason they want me on the show. My imperfections aren't just relatable. They are trending.

As I begin to prep the segment, though, something feels wrong. *Dexter, where are you? I need to talk.* I have to figure out what's wrong.

I get up from the kitchen table where I work and walk outside. I am followed by Luna, our dog. She's an eight-year-old rescue with a pronounced underbite and a sunny disposition that makes it impossible for her to serve as the same kind of sounding board as Dexter did. That's the problem I have with dogs in general: they are way too happy. If I get Luna's leash, she jumps up and down. If I simply walk into the room, her tail begins to thump. Don't get me wrong, sometimes I need the unconditional love of my sweet pup. But how can I have a serious conversation with her?

I watch her sniff around the yard until she tires or grows bored and lies down in the sun. Such contentment is enviable. She is close to fifty-six years old in human years, almost my same age. I am going to turn sixty in four months. I don't feel old. I have been dying my prematurely graying hair since my twenties. And I am fortunate to be in good health. So I don't have any of the usual concerns about reaching this milestone—certainly not as many as the folks at AARP seem to think I have, judging from the amount of mail I get from them.

What bothers me about my life at this stage of the game is that I am not happier. I wish I was as happy being me as Luna is being a dog. This thought hits me like a punch to the gut after I have gone back inside the house. I am in my library, sitting in an obviously oft-used chair against the window. The sunlight streams in over my shoulder, providing warmth and brightness, while I work on a crossword puzzle. This is heavenly.

Until I lose my concentration. I put my pen down. A heaviness grips my heart and slows things down. *Oh hey, anxiety, I thought that was you. You coming for a visit? What do you need this time?* I sigh and look around and think about where I live and how beautiful everything is and how long it has taken me to create this environment exactly the way I want it. This home is my sanctuary. So why is my heart hurting? Why am I anxious?

I feel guilty thinking this given all these blessings. But would I trade my car, swimming pool, and wine cellar for a heart that overflowed with happiness? Yes. Would I trade financial security for it? That scares me, of course, and sounds like the premise of a novel about a woman who renounces all worldly goods and concerns to make a journey that leads her to a true contentment in her soul. But I may not be courageous enough to give up my house, my six-burner Wolf range, my face cream, and my chardonnay. Is there a middle ground?

When Wolfie first learned to talk, he spent one Christmas walking up to anybody and everybody at our house, and asking, "Are you happy?" My sister-in-law put a picture of him on a T-shirt and wrote beneath it, ARE YOU HAPPY? It was a predigital meme. That image popped into my head one day last summer while I was writing in my journal. I wondered what it was like to be truly happy from the inside out.

*What does it feel like to be peacefully happy? I'm really good at putting on a happy face and pretending to be happy, but it never feels like it sinks into my heart and soul.*

*What is missing?*

. . . . . . . . .

"It just can't be about weight anymore," I say.

I am on the phone with the *Today* show producer.

"I have been losing the same ten pounds for fifty years. It can't be the ten pounds. I am tired of that conversation. I have been having it my entire life, and I don't know if it's even relevant. What I want to know is this: How do I love myself the way I am right now? In this body. At this age."

I may never lose the weight. If I could lose it and keep it off, I would. But . . . and it's a big *but* (pun intended) . . . I have spent nearly every day since I was thirteen getting on the scale in the morning and afternoon without ever being happy or satisfied with the number I see. That's more than thirty-two thousand steps on and off the scale ending in disappointment. My journal is a chronicle of frustration and failure. I have recorded my weight every day without ever seeing the right number. Why have I made my happiness contingent on a number that will never satisfy me?

*Enough already.*

This is a change of course for me and a different message to everyone who has followed me on my journey. I meant what I said before, but I feel like I'm finally getting at the truth of the matter. Like so many other people, I have spent most of my life assuming that I have to lose weight and fix myself. It's been a life of denial, criticism, and punishment. I have been chasing a so-called healthy look at the expense of my mental health. I don't want to treat myself that way anymore. I don't want to talk to myself that way anymore.

I'm done with judging myself. I don't want to think in terms of fat or thin. I don't want to look at the scale every day. It's not working, and it's obviously not helping me look in the mirror and see the best version of me at that moment.

I have a whole list of "I don't want tos."

What *do* I want?

I want to be kinder and more accepting of myself.

I want to feel joy inside me.

I want to accept and appreciate myself and recognize the good instead of only seeing what I have always thought of as bad.

I want to stop using the word "bad" to describe myself.

I wouldn't mind getting rid of "fat" and "ugly," too.

I know some days will be harder than others. But I want to remember that I get through them and come out feeling better and stronger.

If I judge myself, I want it to be for the things that matter — am I a generous, loving human being who recognizes the gift of life, starting with my own?

"It's enough already," I tell my *Today* show producer. "I'm going to be sixty years old. I want to get my shit together."

They like this suggestion. The wheels of production turn. Natalie Morales schedules time to interview me at home. I book a flight to New York and prepare for an in-studio chat with Hoda and the gang. Everyone is excited about this shift to something much deeper and more revealing than another diet story.

Once I hang up, I ask myself what I have done. I am someone who hides behind a smile, a joke, a glib "Everything's fine," or a chirpy "It's all good" — even when it isn't, which has been the situation lately. I lost my dad in 2016, then, after doing my best to take care of my mom, she passed away this past June. As a way of managing, I ate myself through the sadness and stress. And now I am worried about Ed and concerned about Wolfie. How am I coping? By trying to perfect my sausage and peppers recipe.

. . . . . . . . .

My interview with Natalie is a tearfest during which I reveal that I feel like I have neglected myself while spending my entire life doing what I think will please everybody else. I have worked since I was twelve, I tell her. Publicly, I have pretended to be the bubbly, upbeat, all-American girl everybody wants to believe I am, but in private, I have rarely thought of myself as anything but a failure. This admission causes me to cry on camera. Later, after the crew has packed up and gone home, I am devastated.

A few days later, I am on the *Today* show set with Hoda and Jenna. Tears flow as I talk about losing my dad and taking care of my mother until we lost her, too, and the other issues that have made the past year or two pretty rough. I open up about turning to food to stifle my emotions and the pain and shame I have felt from gaining back my weight. Admitting this makes me feel vulnerable, but I note that mindfulness expert Brené Brown says that acknowledging your vulnerability is freeing. I joke that I fear a vulnerability hangover coming on.

The strange part of doing this on live television is the way the set turns very small, intimate, and almost private the more I open up to Hoda and Jenna. It's like we're in a safe little bubble. At the same time, I am aware that this is being watched by millions of people, many of whom will no doubt ask why I am willing to bare my soul and dissolve into a blubbery mess while they drink their morning coffee.

But I know others see themselves in me and are helped by these segments. It makes me wonder if my calling is not acting or having my own cooking show but holding myself up as an example of the constant struggle to fix or forgive ourselves for the imperfections that make us all human. Does this mean I am an emotional streaker? Am I an empathy addict? If any of this is true, it should be noted that I am exhausted from it.

And the work has only just begun.

I am eager to get rid of the heavy emotions I have carried around. I want to quit eating my feelings and deal with them in a healthy manner. I want to reset my life.

I want to feel happy and real joy.

. . . . . . . . .

Is it even possible?

I am glad that I called off the diet. As I start the new year, it feels like a weight has already been lifted from my shoulders. Since I am not trying to lose ten pounds, I do not start the day by getting on the scale and setting myself up for disappointment. This is not only liberating, it is also a relief not to hear my inner voice call me a failure.

But it seems stupid to think I can change when I have no long-lasting track record. Eighteen months after giving birth to Wolfie, I went to see a therapist. She asked why I was there. I said I was tired of being angry, then I started to sob.

"I want to be a happy mother," I said. "I want to change."

And here I am almost twenty-eight years later.

Do you know what frustrates me most about that? Ed changed and I didn't. For so long, he was a tortured individual who drank and did drugs as a way of fighting his demons and insecurities. Many times he came offstage angry at some piece of equipment. Or else he was mad at David Lee Roth, who knew exactly how to get under Ed's skin. Even after Wolfie joined the band, Ed had years where his behavior was impossibly cruel. Then he got sober and was back to being the kindhearted soul I fell in love with when I was twenty years old. He is still a gruff, set-in-his-ways, often stubborn man. But there was a lightness to him. And it's still there. Wonderful. Inviting. Irresistible. Happy to be here.

I don't want to go through his same hell to get to that lightness. There has to be an easier way. But I still envy it.

His lightness.

His happy to be here.

. . . . . . . . .

Through the *Today* show, I am introduced to Angie Johnsey, a mind coach who specializes in teaching people how to deal with emotional pain without using food as a crutch. She is a lithe woman with a dancer's build, blonde hair, and a thick Alabama accent. She is gentle and warm. I like her immediately, especially as she nods knowingly when I give her my spiel about how this all started after I said, "Enough already, I don't want to start the year off saying I need to lose ten pounds in order to be happy."

"I never stick to my resolutions, either," she says with a shrug that conveys a refreshing honesty and self-acceptance.

There are three main pillars to the work Angie does: listening to your thoughts, cutting out sugar, and exercising. The last two are obvious. Sugar is addictive and derails your brain from clear thinking and healthy decisions, and moving your body feels good. We spend the most time discussing what to do with the thoughts and emotions that constantly grind me down and overwhelm me. Angie calls this mental consciousness. During a few sessions, she helps me identify the issues giving me the most trouble—anger, sadness, feeling like a failure—and shows me her method for thinking of the mind as a house with various rooms where thoughts can be gathered and organized and addressed.

Otherwise, she explains, it's like walking into a house that's a complete mess. Everywhere you look is a disaster area. It overwhelms you.

I know the feeling.

She encourages me to listen to my thoughts carefully, hear them as part of an ongoing conversation, identify them, and put them in the appropriate room in my brain. The majority go in a Mission Room — those are your practical to-dos, the things I can control (grocery shopping, going to the doctor, finding a new book to read, checking in on a parent, volunteering). The big pie-in-the-sky wishes that aren't easily addressed or accomplished by a single task but are nonetheless important go in the God Room (being happier, worrying about a loved one's health, wanting to fall in love). Then there's the Trash Room — the place for all the self-criticism, doubts, and anxiety (calling myself a failure, seeing only my imperfections).

If ignored, she says, your thoughts only yell louder, bang on the walls, and eventually kick down the door.

Has she been eavesdropping in my head?

A few working sessions and phone calls don't fix my issues, but they open my eyes and give me tools I can use going forward. I tell myself that it's a process. I can't beat myself up forever over old narratives, real or not. I will try to listen to the voices no matter how negative they are, and instead of reacting or overreacting, I will try to understand why they are talking to me and what they want and need, and why they are asking to be heard. What is the little girl who was never heard trying to say? What kind of help does the young woman who was so confused and insecure need? What fears and anger does the grown-up me need to get out?

When I go back on the *Today* show at the end of January, I tentatively report having some breakthroughs. What is refreshing is that these said breakthroughs have nothing to do with weight loss. There is no talk of success or failure. Instead, I describe having experienced several moments at home during which I felt deep inside a genuine lightness of being. As I hear myself talk, I am momentarily struck by what I have just said. "Lightness" is not a word I have ever used in conjunction with myself. But that's exactly what I felt. It was an ease and comfort within me that wasn't there before. Then it was gone.

I want more, dammit.

And I get more — just not in the way I thought.

. . . . . . . . .

It happens a while later.

I lose my wallet. In the grand scheme of things, this is not a big deal. Every day is not always life or death. Sometimes it's more annoying than that.

This is how it goes down: I go to the grocery store in the afternoon and come straight home. I leave my purse in the car, as I normally do, and bring the grocery bags inside. The next morning, I need something in my wallet and walk into the garage to get it. I look in my purse and my wallet isn't there.

The last time this happened to me was about twenty-five years ago. I had taken Wolfie, then about three or four years old, to Toys "R" Us. I had a crazy time putting his fidgety little butt back in his car seat. Distracted, I drove home without realizing my backpack was still in the shopping cart in the parking lot.

That backpack had my life in it: my driver's license, credit cards, bank cards, notes, photos, and my daily calendar/personal diary. I never saw any of it again.

I was very upset, but a part of me fantasized about saying good riddance and starting over with a brand-new ID. Not just height and weight but everything. At the time, my life was not working. Ed and I were in our second year of therapy. I was commuting between Park City and Los Angeles while shooting a miniseries and missing my son. My hair was blonde, my belly button was newly pierced, and the pile of self-help books on my nightstand was mostly unread.

I was *this far* from waving the white flag at the time.

Starting over was an appealing concept.

But my reaction to losing my wallet is entirely different this time. I never think about trading myself in for a different version, not even a skinnier me (well, not very often). When I call the grocery store and the manager confirms that my wallet is in their lost and found, I race to the store to get it back — and get me back.

It is a lesson in disguise.

The joy I want to feel is not so much an end goal as it is a value and an intention that I must choose and realign with over and over again.

# The World's Best Eggs

## MARCH 2020

T IS WOLFIE'S BIRTHDAY, and this is the first one that Ed and I will not celebrate with him. It's the first one the three of us will not be together. My heart aches.

For years, we celebrated Wolfie's birthday and other special occasions with a family dinner at a small Italian restaurant called Il Tiramisu in Sherman Oaks. The end of our marriage did nothing to alter this tradition. After our beloved restaurant closed, we took Wolfie and any friends he wanted to invite to Morton's steakhouse, where I always ordered lobster and a martini, Wolfie enjoyed the salmon, and Ed usually asked for a steak.

But it is March 16, and Los Angeles is under lockdown thanks to the new coronavirus pandemic. We aren't quite sure what this virus means, but it's scary.

Today's *Los Angeles Times* says that "it's time to hunker down." In an effort to slow the spread of this virus, the mayor has issued an emergency order closing restaurants, bars, nightclubs, schools, stores, gyms, and all events of fifty people or more. I am glued to cable news, watching every day with disbelief and an insatiable hunger for information.

I saw disease expert Dr. Anthony Fauci say the worst has yet to come. I also saw President Trump say of the virus, "It's something we have tremendous control of."

Time will tell.

I can't believe this is happening.

Actually, I can. The facts and the science don't lie.

But I don't want to believe it. There are enough problems in the world without adding a worldwide pandemic. These past four years have seemed like a wackadoodle reality TV series, and now it feels like we're building to a cataclysmic ending. I am waiting for Denzel Washington, Liam Neeson, or Keanu Reeves to show up and kick some butt and get us out of this mess.

I am meeting regularly with Angie and working her program. We have our weekly video chats and try to reinforce the ways I can separate my thoughts and emotions. I will catch myself asking where the weight loss is, but I try to do that less. I am trying to get to a place where I look at myself the way Wolfie did when he was a little boy—with pure love.

That's not anything that can be captured in before and after pictures. It's a process I have to practice every day.

I don't let my disappointment about Wolfie's birthday define the entire day. It's out of my control. Even though I am going to miss seeing Wolfie and Ed, who, I learn from Wolfie, is equally bummed, there's nothing I can do about it. I put the negativity in Angie's Trash Room and remind myself that motherhood is something I got wonderfully, blissfully right. Just thinking about it fills my heart with joy.

And there it is, that feeling—pure joy. At this age. In this body.

· · · · · · · · ·

A year after Ed and I split, Wolfie, then twelve years old, inter-viewed Ed and me for a school project. Wolfie and I had moved into the house where I still live. Ed came over, as he still frequently did, and the two of us sat next to each other on the living-room sofa facing Wolfie, who pointed a video camera at us.

I was up first.

"Okay, Mom, tell me about me," he asked. "What was I like as a baby?"

I watched that video recently, so it's fresh in my mind. I spoke nonstop for about twenty minutes, recalling every cute and won-derful thing I remembered, starting with the miraculous feeling I had when my doctor looked up at me in the delivery room, and said, "You have a boy." Then it was Ed's turn. I leaned back and bit my lip as he said a few things. I was icy cold toward him and mad, and now, after watching that video, I'm mad at myself for being that way. My feelings were real. I was upset with Ed for so many things, not the least of which was the egregious lapse in responsi-bility that caused me to finally leave him. He had flown with Wol-fie back to Los Angeles from Park City, where I was working, and he had cocaine on him. But he was sober as Wolfie videotaped us. Was it necessary to still be so angry? Who did it help? What good did it do any of us?

· · · · · · · · ·

Love.

Ed and I always intended to have a family. I miscarried a few years into our marriage, and we put off trying again in order to fo-cus on our careers. By 1990, though, I was ready. After ten years of marriage, we were building our dream house in Coldwater Canyon with enough rooms for us to have three or four children. I was thirty years old and my TV series, *Sydney*, had just been cancelled. I had nothing on the radar. "Let's really try now," I told Ed, and two and a half weeks later I was pregnant.

I was never happier than when I had this new life growing in me. I felt like Wonder Woman at the outset. Then, about six weeks into my pregnancy, I was hit by pretty severe morning sickness that lasted all day and night. I sucked on lemons to combat the nausea, but I told myself that the sickness and all the other changes my body went through were a part of this amazing experience and that I should learn to love it.

I also discovered that the nausea went away when I ate. So I ate. Sandwiches were a favorite. Turkey, muenster, and roast beef on rye. Peanut butter and jelly. Italian subs. Whatever I felt like. It was the first time since adolescence that I let myself eat with impunity. I was finally *allowed* to eat, as if I needed permission. Having been on a diet since I was fifteen years old, I had trained myself to think of food in terms of denial and restriction rather than enjoyment and health. Suddenly, I was free to indulge—and I did. I was like, "Hold the guilt, add the mayo."

I did not, however, ease up on the pressure I put on myself to get motherhood exactly right (whatever that meant). In addition to reading all the books, I asked my mom questions constantly. I wanted to know everything about childbirth and child-rearing, as if I might be missing information. I was full of anxiety. I wanted to do everything perfectly. I didn't want to make any mistakes. Finally, my mom told me to relax.

"You're reading too many books," she said. "You're asking too many questions. You'll be fine. It comes to you naturally."

I was so mad at her for seeming to not understand the way

I prepared. When I got ready for a role, I did a lot of preparation on the character, and made voluminous notes about this person. Even if I forgot my lines, which I did all the time, the work I did let me get to an emotional moment faster and improvise in a way that made sense. It was more than memorizing the script. I had the character down and could handle any changes that were made on the fly.

As I came to learn, my mom was right. There were basics, but motherhood didn't come with a set script. For a new mom like me, it was more important and indeed crucial to understand the character, her backstory, and the challenges she would face going forward. Why did she want to be a mom? What was she doing to be a good mom? Was she prepared for this kind of love? The job was about being able to organize, prioritize, and improvise.

My first clue that this was true should have been Wolfie's refusal to stick to the schedule. I was two weeks past my due date when my doctor insisted that I had waited long enough. I needed to be induced. We set a date: March 16. On the afternoon before, while Ed was in Riverside buying a blue and white Nomad, which happened to have the license plate SHES MAD (fitting for the situation), I enjoyed a bottle of 1972 Chateau Montelena with my parents. My doctor had given me the go-ahead to relax with a glass of wine. That is not an instruction I found in any of the baby books I read, but it should be.

It was essentially the same advice Angie Johnsey gave me thirty years later. Just in a different context.

*Relax.*

*Trust your instincts.*

*Everything will be okay.*

*Motherhood is a long game. Play it that way. This is just the start.*

Later that night, Ed drove me to Saint John's Hospital in Santa Monica, where I went straight to the cafeteria and devoured one of the most delicious grilled cheese sandwiches of my life. That should be another instruction in baby books: have a grilled cheese sandwich.

I was scheduled to be induced at 8 a.m. the next day. My last words to Ed—after I said, "Goodbye, have a good night, I love you"—were "please don't be late."

Guess what?

He was late.

Ed rolled in around 9 a.m. I supposed that was pretty close to eight in rock-star time. By then, I was an hour into my Pitocin drip and was having contractions. He was lucky I wasn't armed. Nine hours later, Ed was holding my hand and trying to coach me through the home stretch. But every time he said, "Push," I smelled peanuts on his breath. I was so hungry and in such discomfort and pain that the smell was amplified. I recognized it immediately, too. It was a PayDay candy bar—my favorite.

I couldn't believe his lack of consideration. How could he?

Very easily, as it turned out.

A few minutes earlier, while I was catching my breath between contractions, he snuck out and scarfed down a PayDay. I had no time to complain more than I did. Finally, at 6:56 p.m., Wolfie arrived, weighing nearly eight pounds and measuring twenty-one inches in length, and Ed switched from a candy bar to a cigar. But the incident was not forgotten. Twenty-seven years later, Wolfie, Ed, and I were celebrating Wolfie's birthday. At dinner, we reminisced and traded stories. Then, as we got ready to order dessert, Ed said he had a present for me. Grinning, he reached into his jacket pocket and pulled out . . . guess what?

A PayDay.

. . . . . . . . . .

When Wolfie was two or three years old, he got in the habit of suddenly breaking away from whatever was occupying him at the moment and running up to me, sometimes bumping into my legs at full speed as if he didn't yet know how to put on the brakes. Then, looking up at me with his big, brown, beautiful, adoring eyes, he would say, "Mama up."

He wanted me to pick him up and give him a hug and a kiss. Every time he did that, I stopped whatever I was doing and obliged. To me, this was motherhood—to pick up my kid and give him a hug and a kiss.

It's also about being a good partner and a decent human being. Our job is to lift each other up.

Most of my issues, I realize, stem from being too focused on myself. I get myself in trouble when left on my own to gaze in the mirror, step on a scale, or sit and ruminate. My brain will seek out the dark clouds and head straight toward them. I'm like the ketjap I let simmer too long at Thanksgiving. I burn.

I have a painting in my library that Wolfie made when he was in kindergarten. At the time, I was working on the miniseries *Night Sins* in Park City. It was a two-month shoot, and even though I flew back and forth most weekends and Ed brought Wolfie up for long weekend visits when I wasn't able to get home, I had never been away from Wolfie that long. I was miserable. He missed me, too.

In his kindergarten class, the teacher asked the students to paint a picture showing what they would do if they had wings. His classmates drew pictures of themselves flying to the candy store or racing birds in their backyard. Wolfie's said, "If I had wings, I would fly to Park City, Utah."

After I saw that, I didn't work for almost five years.

My manager was frustrated and irritated with me for turning down work. Finally, he asked, "What do you do all day?"

I fixed meals for Wolfie: broccoli and fusilli, meatloaf, turkey meatball soup. I volunteered in his classrooms. I needlepointed him a Christmas stocking. I drove him to Little League practices and games and AYSO soccer at the park. A lifelong sports fan, I looked forward to Saturdays when Ed and I set up our folding chairs along the sideline of the soccer field and watched Wolfie's games. I was happy when it was my turn to bring snacks for his team.

My closest friendships today are with the mothers I met when Wolfie started kindergarten. Even his teacher is a friend. We asked each other questions, laughed at our mistakes, and traded tips and tricks. Those friendships became vital to the process of raising my child. I don't think anyone can do it alone—and why would anyone want to?

As our kids got older and went to different schools, our conversations addressed new topics, but the questions, laughter, and tips continued. Occasionally, we helped one another through tears.

Those were the women I turned to for advice and support when Ed wanted Wolfie to go on tour with Van Halen in 2007. At the time, Wolfie was a newly minted sixteen-year-old. I was petrified to let him go. What mother in her right mind would let her son bid sayonara to eleventh grade and tour the world with a hard-rocking band led by his dad who was still, in his early fifties, battling his own demons and abusing alcohol and drugs in a way that made him unpredictable and volatile?

That was the whole reason I left Ed when Wolfie was ten years old. I couldn't let Wolfie see that kind of behavior any longer. I had to protect him.

When he was sixteen, though, how much protecting could I do? How much did he need?

How much had he already seen?

Wolfie, in fact, was the one who came up with the idea of inviting the band's original lead singer, David Lee Roth, back into the group for a reunion tour. He even made the first phone call to David's manager.

The rational part of me knew that this group wasn't the Van Halen of the eighties. Each of the guys—Ed, Alex, and David— were deeply ensconced in their own adult worlds. Most of whatever resemblance they had to the band of legend was onstage, and I do have to say that this part was still legendary. Offstage, they had aches and pains and issues. Ed and I had joint custody of Wolfie, so one or both of us could have put our foot down. But we never brought lawyers into our differences and I wasn't about to start now.

I still roared like a mama bear and gave a list of demands. I insisted that Wolfie have a guardian and a tutor to keep up his schoolwork. I wanted assurance that he would have healthy food. And I wanted carte blanche to come out on the road and travel with them anytime I wanted to. Ed agreed to everything. Wolfie hugged me. Then, as only a teenage boy can do, he reduced all our talks and my concerns to the bare minimum. He said that he was going to have the best time, and he told me not to worry.

Yeah, right.

I had been raised Catholic but had long since lapsed in terms of structured religion. But I had lived in California long enough to develop a recipe for my own spiritual soup. It still included a belief in God, a higher power who accepted collect calls in emergencies. I put in a call and asked God to watch out for my baby. *He's the bass player. The others are on their own.*

During the tour, he experienced the highs of entertaining tens of thousands of people who showed up to love the music and the band. He also witnessed the lows of his dad's struggles onstage and off. It upset me when I saw that he tried to bottle up his feelings the same way that I did. I guess I had done my damage; I couldn't protect him any longer.

We had some very frank talks. He obviously saw things that I had hoped he wouldn't see, and I saw a young man emerging with a big, open, sensitive, forgiving heart.

. . . . . . . . .

March 16, 2020. Wolfie's birthday. At about the time we normally would have been sitting down to a celebratory dinner, I sent Ed a text. "Sending you love on this special day. 💜 What a boy we have."

Ed responded immediately. "Right?? Happy birthday to you too, Val!! 💜"

We have always considered Wolfie's birthday a celebration of the love the two of us shared when we created him and the effort we made to raise him.

The first time I changed Wolfie's poopy diaper, I was so wound up about doing that and everything else right that I burst into tears. The tears went away, but the anxiety didn't. For years, I felt like I was doing so many things wrong. Now I step back and see the amazing adult man Wolfie has become, and I wish I hadn't beaten myself up so much. It's allowed me to do something I rarely do — give credit to myself. I did a pretty good job.

I think of a recent interview he did about his new songs. I had gone over to his house early in the morning to be there in case he needed me. I made soft scrambled eggs, cooking them slowly in a sauce pan on a low flame, adding butter and a splash of olive oil, seasoning with salt and pepper, breaking up the curds, and stirring ever so patiently as if I didn't have to be anywhere all week. As I had learned, fluffy, creamy, delicious scrambled eggs must be pampered to perfection. Wolfie called them the "world's best eggs."

I agreed but for a different reason. My slow cookery allowed me to stick around and eavesdrop on the interviews. When someone asked him how he handled the groupies the first time he went on tour with Van Halen, I stopped stirring and turned so my ear was angled toward him. Without hesitation, he said that he didn't see any groupies. He stayed on the tour bus, he said, and played his video games. Then he texted his mom.

# Soft Scrambled Eggs

Like so much in life, the secret to making the world's best eggs is to take your time. Go slowly. The day is ahead of you. Enjoy it.

| | | | |
|---|---|---|---|
| 3 | tablespoons unsalted butter | 1 | teaspoon kosher salt |
| 1 | tablespoon of olive oil | ¼ | teaspoon freshly ground black pepper |
| 8 | large eggs | | |

Heat the butter and oil in a nonstick skillet over medium-low heat. Once the butter is melted, add the eggs into the pan.

Use a rubber spatula or whisk to break the yolks and scramble the eggs. Stir the eggs continuously until small curds start to form.

Season the eggs with the salt and pepper.

Continue stirring the eggs with a rubber spatula over a low heat until the eggs are soft but solidified, about 10 to 15 minutes. Turn the heat off. Serve warm.

**Serves** 3 to 4 people

# My Wallabees

MARCH 2020

WANT TO APOLOGIZE FOR still talking about my weight. By now, the script has to be tired and boring. It is for me. Nothing is drearier or more unproductive than the well-worn path from my bed to the scale, and yet it is the rare day that I can avoid that route. I need someone to put up a detour sign. Just pee, wash your face, and go straight to the coffee maker.

TMI?

Sorry.

No matter how old we get, I think everyone struggles with this question of what to hang on to and what to discard from the past. These can be habits, routines, or material things. It starts when our parents put our favorite stuffed animal on a shelf instead of letting us sleep with it or tell us to quit sucking our thumb, explaining, "You don't need that anymore," and we go from there— or we don't.

I know people in their fifties who still keep their baby blankie nearby. Forty-five years later, I still wake up and head for the scale.

*Enough already.*

I'm trying.

But the stuff we hang on to is not all bad.

A friend recently asked me if I felt grown-up and I answered without hesitation. Yes, I feel like a grown-up. I don't feel finished—and I don't know if I ever want to feel that way. I want to believe that I am still learning, developing, and acquiring new insights, tricks, and wisdom. In other words, I am still growing—or trying to. But I definitely feel like a grown-up.

It happened gradually. I did not feel mature when I bought my first house at nineteen, and my twenties were a disaster. I am ashamed of most everything I did and said back then. The turning point was Wolfie. Giving birth to him was what caused me to grow up. I was thirty and suddenly responsible for a new life.

Well, not suddenly. I had nearly ten months of pregnancy to adjust. No drugs, no partying, no kooky diets, no crazy high heels. I remember that voice of God in my head—or maybe it was my mother: *You're having a baby. Grow up.* Pushing a fully formed human being out of my body did the trick. If that doesn't get your attention, nothing will. I remember telling *People* magazine how Ed and I brought our newborn home, sat on the sofa with him, looked at each other, and asked, "What now?"

I learned.

It took Ed a bit longer.

Now I am nearly sixty and Ed is sixty-five. I know how that happened. But how did it happen so quickly? Where did the time go? The time—that's really the thing we all try to hang on to, whether it's the yearbooks we refuse to throw out, the plastic surgery some people get, or the habits and the hurt that are so hard to shed. I can't believe I am the age I am now and still dealing with thoughts and issues that plagued me as a teenager. Then again, I will never part with some things from my past.

As Shakespeare wrote—or maybe it was Marie Kondo—to toss or not to toss, that is the question.

· · · · · · · · ·

I still have my favorite pair of Wallabees from seventh grade. I think they are officially called Clarks desert boots. They are tucked somewhere in my closet. They cost one hundred sixty dollars now. Back then, I think they were around twenty-three dollars, which was considered expensive. I don't even know if they were marketed for women and girls then. They were sold as crepe-soled hiking boots for men.

When I got mine in the seventies, we were only a few years past the school dress code's being modified to allow girls to wear pants to school. If I remember correctly, girls were *allowed* to wear pants only on Fridays at first. A year later, we could wear them every day. Good grief. The idiocy of girls having a dress code. Don't get me started.

In 1975 I was cast as Barbara Cooper, the youngest of two daughters being raised by a divorced mom, on Norman Lear's new sitcom *One Day at a Time.* Bonnie Franklin starred as the mom, and Mackenzie Phillips played my older sister. It featured Pat Harrington as our apartment building's superintendent. The show broke new ground in that it was the first sitcom about a single woman raising children on her own. It changed my life. I literally grew up on the show and in front of the entire country.

It was such a different era. *One Day at a Time* was among top-rated series that also included *All in the Family, Laverne & Shirley, The Bionic Woman, Sanford and Son,* and *Happy Days.* In the days when there were only three major channels, twenty-five to thirty million people tuned in each week.

One week that first season, I wore my Wallabees on an episode. With either jeans or a skirt, it was a good look. More than that, it was my look. Straight out of my closet.

Every time I clean out my closet, I keep those shoes. Whether I have moved, decided to downsize, or grown bored with the choices, those Wallabees remain on the shelf. They are an old friend I check in with once every few years. Just a quick conversation.

"Hey, there you are. Are you good?"

"I'm good. How are you?"

"I'm good, too. Okay, see you later."

I was starting Robert Frost Junior High School when I got them. Every year, before school started, my mom bought us new clothes. My brothers got a new pair of pants and a couple of T-shirts, and I got a new outfit, and we picked out a new pair of shoes at Thom McAn. I got the Wallabees. They were soft and clean and exactly what I wanted.

I was an alternate cheerleader that year. I remember wanting to fit in. Of course, I had no idea that everybody else had the same fears and anxieties about being accepted and popular and wanting to fit in. I picked out the Wallabees because the cool kids had them and I was going for cool by association. I was never cool, and as I recall, one girl was always excluded from the in-crowd, and when I was that girl, it sucked. But that was rare. I was a spunky, fun-loving kid who played sports with my brothers and laughed often and loudly.

Those shoes sit on my shelf as a reminder of what it felt like to be happy through and through and, even more important to me right now, that it was possible.

· · · · · · · · · ·

My father was a pack rat, maybe even a borderline hoarder. But he was organized and very proficient with a label maker.

Me, not so much.

I have been talking to Ed about returning a pair of his Dr. Martens boots that somehow ended up at my house. They are on one of the bookshelves in my library, and it seems like they have been there forever. I don't remember when or how they appeared. He must have taken them off and forgotten them one time when he was here. I know he loves his Dr. Martens. This pair is black and heavily worn. One boot even has tape wound around it. I keep mentioning that I want to return them, but either I forget or he is in the hospital.

"I'll just wait till I can go up to your house," I tell him.

"That's fine," he says.

"They're just sitting on a shelf in my library," I say.

"I wonder how they got there." He laughs.

"Me, too."

I think both of us know that the odds of my returning them are slim. I can look around me and see other things that I will never part with. Like the wooden high chair I used for Wolfie, and the old wine cart that my mom treasured and used for parties when I was growing up. I also have all my scripts from *One Day at a Time* and *Hot in Cleveland*. There is a lamp from my first house that still works and the gorgeous old piano that I also bought for that house. It's broken and missing keys, and I have been told it is not worth the money to fix it, but one day I will turn it into book-shelves or an art piece. It ain't going anyplace without me.

On a shelf in my dining room's breakfront hutch, I have a small collection of blue delft miniature houses. Ed and I got them on our first trip to Amsterdam, where we looked up his family roots. It was a phenomenal trip. The miniatures were giveaways in the first-class cabin of KLM airlines. They were beautifully made and filled with liquor. I remember putting them in my bag to keep as mementos of the trip. When we got home, they went on the shelf, where they have sat ever since.

But they haven't gone untouched. One day about fifteen years ago, I was looking at them, reminiscing about the trip, and I wondered how the booze inside them tasted—if it was still even good after all these years. I picked up one, removed the cork, bottomed up, and . . . nothing. It was empty. What? I picked up another. And another. All six, though still corked, were empty. I made a call. Sure enough, Ed drank them a few years before I got to them.

I know I can't keep everything. Though it's rare, once something doesn't fill a need or spark a warm emotion, it's gone. Just the other day I threw out a little magnet on my refrigerator that said, MIR-ACLES HAPPEN. KEEP THE SKINNY JEANS. I wish my scale were next. It's unlikely, but the batteries in it died the other morning and maybe that's a sign.

. . . . . . . . .

I am in my office when Wolfie comes over to the house and calls my cell phone to see if I am there. I still remember the sound of his voice when he walked in the house after school and yelled, "MA!" *What happened to yelling,* I think, as I answer my phone. I ask if he wants to come down and hang out. He politely declines and says that he has just stopped by to spend time with the cats.

Even though he's allergic, he comes over to play with them whenever he has the urge. I am happy whenever that urge strikes, which is frequently.

About an hour later, I walk upstairs and see him through the window. He's curled up on the sofa in the den, petting Bubba and Beau, the two cats I inherited from my parents. My rock star is still a little boy at heart. He looks like he did when he was a kid.

I like that he is not giving that up, and by that, I mean the com-fort of coming home and lying on the couch even though he is an adult. It is a feeling all of us need. I bet I could do a gangbuster business if I opened a store where people could come in, lie on a couch for an hour, and have a gray-haired *bubbe* tuck them under a blanket and tell them that everything is going to be okay. Just shut your eyes and rest.

Of course, that's also called therapy.

. . . . . . . . .

I could use some counseling now. I have a photo shoot in two days, and the stylist for the shoot has dropped off a bunch of clothes for me to try on. I don't want to try them on or do the shoot, period. I am in a mood where I would rather pull on a T-shirt and call it a day. Sometimes I like these shoots; it's fun to get dressed up in fancy clothes and be fussed over by a hairstylist and makeup artist. Other times, I feel like the camera lens is a microscope zeroing in on the flaws and places I am trying to ignore. This is one of those days.

I am definitely not feeling the joy. I step in front of the mirror and see places on my body that remind me of the junk drawer in the kitchen, that drawer everyone has where things pile up and collect no matter how often it is cleaned and curated. Like the mystery of the one missing sock in the dryer, the junk drawer defies logic. Maybe that's the origin of the phrase "junk in the trunk."

Whatever.

I get anxious. I go for a walk. I have tea. I page through magazines. I read. After a while, I pour myself a glass of wine, sit outside, and try to meditate as I watch the sun glide in slow motion over the far western hills of the valley to wherever it lands on the other side of the Pacific. By then, I am definitely calmer but still engaged in a debate with my more insecure, critical self. Why didn't I go on a diet and lose five pounds? Ten would have been perfect. If I had lost ten, I wouldn't be torturing myself like this.

Then I hear myself, and think, *Oh my God, I am truly insane. I can't hear this song one more time.* I do as Angie has advised. I acknowledge it, understand what it is trying to tell me and how it is trying to protect me in its own twisted way, then I say no thank you and Marie Kondo those voices.

That doesn't make me any thinner. Neither will it make me any more comfortable when I get in front of the camera in two days. But it does stop the chatter and allows me to think rationally. I tell myself that the public already knows what I look like and that losing ten or fifteen pounds might help my knees but it won't affect my smile. I will also be surrounded at the shoot by people I trust whose only goal will be to make me look good. So . . . STFU.

Later that night, I log on to Google Maps and look up the first house Ed and I shared before we were married. It was a cute little New Orleans–style three-story place in the hills with a nice view. I remember fans coming by at all hours after word got out that Ed was living there. People drove by all night with their radios blasting Van Halen, honking their car horns and yelling, "Eddie. Eddie, we love you." I used to think, *Can't you love him in the afternoon?*

Then I look at my childhood homes in Delaware and Michigan and California. I have done this a few times in the recent past as a way of connecting the dots. Where I thought I would see nothing but nostalgic street views and trees that have matured beyond recognition, I instead find memories that let me time travel with a great big smile on my face. I picture myself running through fields, getting stung by a bee, and jumping off the old wooden dock into Walters Lake. I see my dad shoveling snow off the lake so I can go ice-skating. I hear myself laughing as I run around the backyard in cutoffs and bare feet while waiting for my dad to take hot dogs off the grill. And I see myself putting on my Wallabees.

# Nonnie's Rolling Pin

### APRIL 2020

THERE ARE A FEW minutes of confusion after I see my latest text message. "Do you have some time? I have a fun idea. Let me know, G."

Before I even open up my calendar, I have a question: Who is G? I have no idea who this person is or how G got my phone number.

It turns out that G is Food Network star chef Giada De Laurentiis, and she wants me to join her and fellow star chef Alex Guarnaschelli in a Zoom-only special called *Three Italian Chicks Helping a Home Cook*. I am in, no matter what the idea.

I feel like the cool kids have invited me to hang out with them. I can't wait. Then, of course, the anxiety hits. Can I do it? Am I really going to be able to contribute? Or will I be exposed as a fraud?

I don't know Giada well. We haven't spent a ton of time with each other so I would still call myself more of a fan than a friend. She is awesome and her talent and knowledge intimidates me. After getting her degree in social anthropology at UCLA, she studied at Le Cordon Bleu, worked with Wolfgang Puck, and opened her own catering business. And, yes, on top of all that intelligence and talent, she is also that naturally beautiful.

Alex, whom I know a little better, is that way, too. I adore her. Her mother was a cookbook editor, and after graduating from Barnard College—where she majored in art history—Alex worked in some of the best restaurants in France, New York, and Los Angeles before heading up the kitchen at New York's acclaimed Butter restaurant.

Beyond last names with multiple syllables, both of these women share something that I think is essential to their success: a genuine passion for food and turning it into something delicious and memorable for others to enjoy. When I am around them, I am not surprised that they do what they do and are so good at it.

If multisyllabic last names were the only requirement to join this exclusive club, I would be a shoo-in and not feel so immediately insecure after I speak with Giada and find out that the three of us will surprise a Food Network fan and help her make something sumptuous from ingredients she already has in her refrigerator and pantry. "It will be fun," Giada says.

I am sure it will be for her and Alex. As for me, I will have to put myself through the mental gymnastics and imaginary freak-outs of hoping I don't say the wrong thing.

Other than that, I am fine.

I did not ever envision hosting my own TV cooking show and sharing tips with these top-tier foodies. It is one of the happy accidents of my life, though it may not be as much of an accident as I used to think. I spent most of my life on a diet; avoiding food; categorizing foods as good or bad, safe or disastrous; restricting my intake; denying myself the pleasure of eating; refusing social invitations if I felt I couldn't *afford* a meal; fearing the bread basket at restaurants; and endlessly calculating calories. There are ninety in an apple, zero in a stalk of celery, five hundred sixty-three in a Big Mac, and two hundred in your average gin martini (give or take depending on the number of olives in your glass).

How was I supposed to let all that go and immerse myself in a life of food? But maybe it is more interesting to wonder how I got to that point and what happened when I did.

Before I incorporated a monkish regimen of restriction and punishment, I thought food was the way you expressed love. Until I was eight years old, I lived with my parents and three brothers in Claymont, Delaware. My father's family was nearby, and we spent countless afternoons and evenings at my Aunt Adeline's house, where she, my Nonnie, and the other women in the family gathered in her basement kitchen and made pasta while trading the latest news and gossip.

To me, that was our family. My grandmother and her *cappelletti in brodo* and her gnocchi and homemade bread. I can't picture her without also seeing that flour-filled counter, the giant mixing bowls, and her wooden rolling pin, which she employed with varying degrees of effort, sometimes leaning into it with all her might and other times moving it over the dough with deftness and delicacy, as if she were wielding a magic wand; then, voilà, there were mounds of newly pinched pasta, broth simmering in a pan, and the scent of garlic wafting through the air. And we all were eventually called to the table because dinner was finally ready.

Then we moved to Clarkston, Michigan, then to Los Angeles, where my father went to work at the new General Motors plant there. I was eleven years old. At school, I met a girl who acted in commercials, and I went home and told my mother I wanted to act. Because I was extremely shy, she didn't believe me. But something pushed me. At twelve, I got my first job on a JCPenney commercial. From then on, I was in a world where looks and size mattered. Everyone had their own idea of beauty, and no one was ever happy with their looks, including me. My idea of a meal went from gnocchi to no thank you.

I am simplifying here, but it's the truth when I say that I didn't eat again until 2010 — and by eat, I mean enjoy sitting down at the table for a meal without spoiling it by overseasoning it with guilt. That's a long time to go without something that was a true pleasure and a passion waiting to be discovered, embraced, nurtured, and shared.

· · · · · · · · ·

It was January 2010, and I had a speaking engagement at the oldest theater in Wilmington. My parents traveled back to Delaware with me and we had a little family reunion at my Aunt Adeline's house. The basement that held so many memories for me was intact and unchanged from the way I remembered it forty-plus years ago. I loved that. It was like entering a time machine. I walked downstairs into my childhood's happy place.

A smile instantly appeared on my face. My aunt already had a pot of *cappelletti in brodo* on the stove. My grandmother's recipe had become her recipe. I walked straight over to the pot and inhaled. The aroma was instantly familiar and sublime.

"I have way more in the freezer," Adeline said.

I opened the nearby freezer the way I did when I was little. Inside were bags and bags of her pasta. When she made it, she made a ton. All you have to do is pour broth over it and you have a meal. This was my version of comfort food and exactly what I needed. I was hungry. Starving, in fact. I had spent all of 2007 losing forty pounds on Jenny Craig. Two years later, I lost another ten and fit into a teeny-weeny bikini two weeks before I turned forty-nine.

Then I reconnected with my Aunt Adeline's *cappelletti in brodo*. With the first spoonful, I thought God had finally heard me and answered my prayers.

I was reunited with my people—and my pasta. I wanted more. I told my husband Tom that we needed to get out our suitcases and check our passports. I wanted to go to Italy. My family's roots were there. Stories were passed down, not in great detail and not always accurately, but they were told and treasured. I had dreamed of traveling there, eating there, seeing the art, appreciating the history, and communing with the spirit of the people and the warmth of the land that I had heard and read so much about all my life. I had traveled around the world with Van Halen, visiting Japan, England, France, Spain, Germany, Sweden, Brazil, Venezuela, and Mexico. Somehow I had missed Italy. How did that happen?

Everyone has these kinds of holes in their life résumés. They get filled over time—when the time is right and we are ready. I was finally ready. I knew I had to go.

When I travel, I normally don't do much planning other than picking a hotel. I usually go out of town for work, so things like transportation and meals are taken care of. It's rare that I have time to slip out for a show or a museum, though I do like to wander around New York when I have the time and I try to find at least one good restaurant. Italy was different. Once Tom and I committed to the trip, I planned as if I were putting together a dinner party. The hotel was the table setting. The restaurants, museums, historical sites, and wineries I wanted to visit were the ingredients needed to make the various courses. I spoke with friends who had been there. I looked at books. We contacted a guide. We created a schedule with time left open for spur-of-the-moment adventure or indulgent afternoon naps. As with any vacation, I not only wanted to get away from myself, I also wanted to leave space to discover or rediscover parts of myself that I had neglected or ignored for far too long.

The long flight was more enjoyable than I expected. I had my bag of magazines, snacks, water, and the book I was reading at the time. I also scrolled through the available movies. But once we got past the initial anxiety of takeoff, I relished the hours I had of being disconnected from daily life. My phone wasn't going to ring. I didn't have any appointments. I wasn't going to spend a minute in traffic or a second worrying that I was running late. It was as if I had packed up all the things that normally consume me and put them in the overhead storage bin.

I stared out the window at the clouds, something I don't do often enough. It reminded me of when my mother, a wonderful artist, looked at a blank canvas before starting a new painting and thought about all the possibilities ahead of her. Eventually, the skies gave way to patches of land.

"That's Europe," Tom said.

"Where are we eating tonight?" I asked.

"Somewhere down there," he said.

"Oh, you know what?" I smiled. "I made a reservation for two at this little place in Rome. Wanna go with me?"

· · · · · · · · ·

Actually, I didn't have reservations. Our hotel was located in the heart of Rome near the Spanish Steps. Although we arrived late at night, we were wide awake. Unlike LA, Rome seemed wide awake, too. After checking into our room, we hurried outside and joined the crowds on the sidewalk. It was the ten o'clock hour and people were just heading to dinner as we intended to. But first we wanted to find the Trevi Fountain.

As a water source, the Trevi Fountain dated back to 19 BC, but it didn't become the ornate attraction we wanted to see until the mid-1700s. Unfortunately, we couldn't find it. The streets confused us. Our GPS said we were close, closer, and eventually right on top of it, but we couldn't see it. We kept getting more and more lost until finally, at the point we were ready to give up because the supposedly short walk felt more like fifteen miles and I was starving, we turned the corner and there it was.

So many travelers say that sometimes you have to get lost to find what you're looking for, and I suppose that can be true. To me, our situation was more about working through frustrations, letting go of the stress, and sticking with the mission. It made looking for pizza afterward even more important than it already was, and the restaurant we stumbled into on our own, La Bruschetta, was so friggin' good.

It was a little place right around the corner from our hotel. We had a simple caprese salad and two thin-crust pizzas that tasted unlike any pizzas I had ever had. I suppose that was because I was eating them in Rome. It was more than just the water. It was the city, the country, the magic of Italy. I had the most amazing night's sleep. In the morning, after a leisurely coffee, we ventured back out into the city. In the daylight, Rome was even more remarkable and beautiful. The city's complexion changed with the light. Yellows turned to gold, then to umber. It was like being in a movie.

The entire city was built on layers of history as we saw when we visited the Coliseum, the Pantheon, the Forum. The Borghese museum's paintings provided a warm-up to the Vatican museums. I have never doubted that looking at great art can be a transcendent and spiritual experience, and Michelangelo's Sistine Chapel and works by Raphael, da Vinci, Caravaggio, Giotto, and others filled my soul. My neck hurt from constantly looking up and twisting around to make sure I didn't miss anything.

My favorite spot in the Vatican was the Gallery of Maps. The room is filled with frescos showing the Italian peninsula. I thought about all the people who must have walked around, taken measurements, and made sketches, and I realized that I was, along with everyone else, participating in this timeless, endless search for direction. I had left home having just been cast in a new TV series called *Hot in Cleveland*, so I wasn't consciously wondering about a next job, where my career was going, whether I was still viable in Hollywood at fifty years old, or if I wanted to do something else with my life — the things that sometimes popped up when I went too long between jobs.

Was there ever going to be a new chapter?

Was I doing what I was supposed to do? I remembered reading a story about an actress who gave up her career to become a nun. I was intrigued by someone who felt such a strong calling. Ed was that way with music. A piano prodigy as a child, he had switched to guitar by age twelve and his relationship with his instrument and music in general only deepened as he got older. It poured out of him. He couldn't not play.

I can't say that I felt the same way about acting. The process made me anxious and I never felt like I was that good at it. I occasionally wondered if I was supposed to do it my entire life. Maybe something else would enrich my life in ways acting didn't. Statistics show that most people change careers a handful of times during their working lives. My father changed jobs but not careers. Ed had only one job. Giada and Alex had numerous jobs, but they were all related to the same passion, cooking. But my friend and former costar Mackenzie Phillips, who struggled with drug addiction much of her life, has spent at least ten years saving lives as a substance-abuse counselor.

All the clichés are true, I suppose. You do what makes you happy, and what makes you happy is generally something you love.

Do I love acting? I don't know. Sometimes.

When it's the right part, yes, I do. I love it.

At that moment, I was in Italy and I knew two things for sure: I loved food, and I was hungry.

For lunch, our guide took us to a little place he knew. My heart sank when we got there and found that the door was locked. I saw it was about two-thirty, so we were arriving when this city takes an afternoon break or *riposo*. Our guide put his hand up. Not to worry. He rapped on the door. The older woman who ran the restaurant peeked out the window, unlocked the door, greeted him with a hug and kisses, and motioned us inside.

It was like walking into my grandmother's house. It smelled like her house after she had been cooking all day. The rich aroma of butter and garlic is a language all its own, one that's universally understood. When I die, I want to be hermetically sealed in this fragrance, Profumo di Italian Cooking.

The lunch was amazing. We had pasta *e fagioli*, pasta carbonara, and a plain green salad. Afterward, while on our way to the Forum, we stopped for a coffee. I ordered a cappuccino with a shot on the side, like I do at home. The barista remained motionless except for a slight shake of his head, telling me no — no cappuccino. In the afternoon, custom called for a single espresso or, more appropriately, a *caffè*.

The next night's dinner fell short of expectations and it was a serious bummer. We ate at a Michelin-starred restaurant that was highly recommended. It was our one big splurge the entire trip and my pasta *alle vongole* was a bust. This is a dish for which Italy is renowned and a favorite of mine. It's simple: butter, garlic, chili, white wine, tomatoes, clams, and pasta. What's not so simple is the deft touch that turns these simmering ingredients into a delicate ballet of briny, buttery, garlicky perfection when they hit the tongue.

So I was disappointed. I said something like, "This can't be happening," which admittedly was bratty on my part. But my expectations were very high for the ten days we were going to be in Italy.

"It's okay," Tom said. "We'll eat again tomorrow."

"I know, I know," I said. "But you only get so many meals in life —and in Italy. Make them all good."

As those words came out of my mouth, they sounded funny and childish. They also reminded me of Ed, who once told me, "You only get so many bottles of liquor in life and I've already gone through mine."

. . . . . . . . .

After bidding goodbye to our favorite waiter at La Bruschetta, the little pizza place we went to the first night and returned to twice more before departing Rome, we ventured to Florence. We began our visit with the Uffizi and the Accademia, taking in Michelangelo's *David* and Botticelli's *The Birth of Venus*, Ghiberti's *Gates of Paradise*, and more from da Vinci and Raphael and other all-stars of the Renaissance until finally I was overwhelmed by all these miracles of human artistry.

After hours of sharing my appreciation for these works of art, I literally ran out of words and decided it was okay to express my reverence with a sated quiet. I even got a little misty eyed from everything I had seen. At that point, we were in the Piazza del Duomo. I couldn't go one step farther and sat down. I needed to catch my breath, rest my legs, drink some water, and feel the sun on my face.

I knew I was reviving when I began to calculate what time we would return to our hotel so I could order an Aperol Spritz, my late-afternoon reward for hiking thousands of miles through museums. After checking my watch, I looked over at Tom and asked the most pressing question of the day: "Where are we eating tonight?"

We ended up at Sostanza, an old trattoria—and by old, I mean it opened in 1869—where we ate—no, make that devoured—their signature dish, butter chicken. It sounds even better in Italian: *petti di pollo al burro*. One bite was all it took for me to pronounce it deserving of its fame and amazing in every sense of the word. It was also deceptively simple to prepare: two chicken breasts are dredged in flour and braised in butter. *Mmm*, just divine.

We ordered more off the menu, but my brain went blotto after the chicken. It was like getting high thirty years earlier. I saw cosmic significance in the taste. I wanted to know if it was wrong to compare it to *David*. Both left me awestruck.

The next day we visited a winery in San Gimignano before returning to Florence for one more day of exploration. Then we headed to Venice. I wanted to go there for a few reasons, starting with the most obvious: Why not go? It's Venice. It's stunning, historic, romantic, and a place where you arrive and immediately know it's special and unique. The other reason I wanted to go was personal. My parents had visited there, and I had grown up hearing their adoring reminiscences of that trip. Already in love, it was the place where they fell in love again.

I adored Venice from the moment I cast my eyes on this waterlogged city. I understood why people said that it seemed to float. The city gave me the sense of not just stepping back in time but also of being magically cast inside a canvas where the foreground of people was constantly being updated against a background painted by the Old Masters. We hopped on a water bus, meandered along the canals, and ended up in St. Mark's Square, where I had the most startling and liberating thought of the trip. After nearly an entire week in Italy, no one had recognized me.

I had spent practically my whole life walking around with blinders on because everyone seemed to know me. But I was anonymous here. I had removed the blinders and was enjoying where I was, and taking everything in, and not feeling like I had to hide. Unlike I did back home, I wasn't missing anything.

It made me wonder how much of my reality was skewed or just plain wrong because of all the things I had blocked out and how much of it was colored by the limited view I permitted myself to see.

. . . . . . . . .

I fell in love with Venice all over again the next day because of something that happened to us every time we stepped outside. Whether we were on our way to St. Mark's Campanile, the Rialto Bridge, or lunch, we got lost. We had a map, but we had no idea where we were going. There seemed to be two directions in Venice—up and water. Everything else was open to debate. Our hotel concierge assured us that this was normal, even desired; he sounded like a therapist when he said, "Don't worry about going anywhere. Just wander and have fun."

Was that where the word "wanderlust" came from—the love of wandering?

We took his advice and promptly had no idea where we were. And that's when I concluded that no one else did, either. Nearly everyone I saw was either lost or holding a map and trying to figure out which way to go on those crazy, confusing Venetian streets. Our fellow travelers were like us, casting about for nonexistent signs while expressing cautious hopefulness. Maybe we were going in the right direction. But if not, who cares, we're in Venice.

People stopped strangers and asked for help. Locals, seeing people struggling with their maps, paused and offered advice and directions. I thought this was incredible to experience, because I am one of those people who can't bring myself to ask for help. I have to be past the point of desperation to wave the white flag, which is stupid, and even then, I have trouble asking for assistance. I think a lot of people are like this—lost, confused, and looking for directions but too scared or embarrassed or ashamed to ask for help.

But in Venice, everyone had granted themselves permission to be confused, even lost. They didn't get all wound up about not knowing all the answers and take their frustrations out on other people. It was okay. All of us eventually found where we wanted to go or we stumbled on something else equally good . . . or even better.

That's how Tom and I ended up having the best dinner of our entire trip. On our second day in Venice, we had gotten lost while meandering through side streets and around canals to look for the perfect out-of-the-way place for lunch. Nothing grabbed us until we spotted a plate of cannoli in the window of a tiny restaurant down an alley. I wasn't even sure it was a restaurant. It might have been a bakery.

We walked in and saw three people eating lunch at a table. They were the only people in the room: two Sicilian guys—the chef and his brother—and a woman, the waitress, who was their friend.

The brother got up and greeted us. I asked if we could get lunch.

"No, no, apologies," he said in heavily accented English. "We are closed."

"But the cannolis," I said, pointing to the window. "I saw them. They look amazing."

"Come back," he said.

"Tonight?"

"Yes, come back tonight." He smiled.

"Eight o'clock?" I said.

"We will see you then."

We managed to somehow find the restaurant again and show up on time. The place was crowded. It was filled with the thick aroma of an Italian kitchen. I knew we were in the right place. I saw that there was a small front room and a slightly larger room in back. I also glimpsed the kitchen, which was minuscule; it looked barely large enough for the chef to move around in. The chef's brother greeted us warmly and showed us to a table. We ordered wine, and I said, "I want to try your pasta *alle vongole*. Other than that, please bring us anything you want to make."

For the next two and a half hours, they kept bringing the most amazing things to eat and taste. Between bites, we learned their stories: the two brothers dreamed of opening a restaurant in Venice and moved from their home in Sicily. I didn't dare ask why they picked this sinking city; it seemed obvious. One of them had a gift for cooking, the other knew business, and both of them had inherited their mother's passion for feeding people. They found this little place and brought their friend to serve the food.

While we were there, I never saw them stop smiling. I told them about my Italian roots, my Nonnie's pasta, and my Aunt Adeline's *cappelletti in brodo* that inspired this trip. It was clear that food was important to all of us, including me. But we weren't talking about eating it as much as we were discussing how to prepare it, and I didn't mention a word about the thing that connected me to food back home: my Jenny Craig diet. I was in the midst of that diet before our trip, but here in Italy, I set it aside and actually forgot about it. I traded restriction for enjoyment.

We sipped some deliciously strong grappa and traded thoughts about choosing ingredients, preparing, and eventually serving the food—the best part, they said, as the brother who was the chef patted his heart.

"Real cooking is about love," I said.

We toasted to *amore*.

· · · · · · · · ·

To be honest, I may have felt like I had some wiggle room to eat while I was in Italy because of all the weight I had lost on Jenny Craig, but once I was back home, I came to another conclusion: I loved food and, more important, I was allowed to love it. I had just experienced ten days where it was okay to enjoy meals.

I tried to figure out why I had been able to not just enjoy my meals and love food but also eat whatever I wanted without getting on a scale once and still feel comfortable not just in my clothes but also in my skin. I didn't weigh myself until I got home. I was shocked that I hadn't gained any weight during the entire trip. What was actually more shocking was that I hadn't spent every day in Italy obsessing about what I ate. I hadn't spent my days stalking the pantry or the refrigerator in a constant test of my self-control, then browbeating myself when my blood sugar plummeted and my willpower inevitably followed.

In Italy, we walked everywhere. I didn't snack. I didn't sit in front of the TV with a bag of junk food because I was bored or angry or frustrated. I ate meals. I enjoyed those meals. I didn't once sit down and think, *This will be my cheat day.* I savored every bite that went into my mouth. In the weeks that passed after we were back home, I frequently thought of the two brothers who ran their little restaurant in Venice and the way they smiled throughout their busy night. I sensed that this joy came from someplace deep inside them, and I wanted that for myself.

It took me another decade of fighting myself to truly understand what that meant and how to try to find that joy within myself, but a spark was lit. I wanted to cook. I had always loved cooking for Ed and Wolfie, and learning new recipes from my mom and Mrs. Van Halen and my group of close women friends. At the time, we were all talking about *The Silver Palate Cookbook*. It had come out in the late eighties, I think, but it was enjoying a resurgence of popularity.

When my manager asked what I wanted to do next, I answered impulsively—or maybe intuitively. Regardless, it was real.

"I would love to do a cookbook," I said, thinking about how much I enjoyed being in the kitchen.

There was no guarantee that I could do it or that anyone would want a book of recipes from me, but I knew I had to try. I mentioned it to my parents. My mom sent me some of her tried-and-true recipes—favorites of mine and Wolfie's. Then one day a package arrived in the mail. Inside was a rolling pin and a card from my father: "This belonged to your grandmother. She used it to roll out her pasta dough when you were a little girl and even when I was a little boy. Now, sweetheart, it's your turn."

It turned out that my Nonnie's rolling pin had been in my mom's kitchen. When I asked why no one had offered it to me before, my mom matter-of-factly said that she never thought I needed it until now. Oddly enough, she was right. Her timing was impeccable.

# Love Cake

## SUMMER 2015

M Y MOTHER WANTED TO contribute to my cookbook. She was unusually effusive. I had the proof in my hand: a large manila envelope with half a dozen recipes inside. These included ones for lasagna and chicken cacciatore and also her spaghetti and meatballs, a staple from my childhood, and for a meat ragù, which my mother noted was a recipe my Nonnie had handed down to her.

The thing I realized about the recipes I got from my grandmother and mother was that neither woman ever consulted a recipe when she cooked, at least not that I saw. So if I wanted to follow one of their recipes, I had to improvise and figure out what tasted good to me.

As I have since learned, there are many good and necessary reasons for creating and following recipes exactly, especially when writing a cookbook, but there is also something to be said about adding a bit of yourself to anything. Follow the basics, then season to taste. That in and of itself is a life motto. Season to taste. Put your toes over the diving board. Step off the path and find your own way.

The recipes my mom sent put a smile on my face. I appreciated her eagerness to contribute and help. She loved to cook; it was central to our family life when I was growing up, whether she was running out to the grocery store for something she forgot, making one of her twice-weekly shopping trips with a long list in hand, preparing a family dinner as she did nightly, or fixing appetizers for my dad's poker nights.

A family of six goes through a lot of food. I don't know that my mom and I ever talked about how she managed and planned our lunches and dinners. Nor do I remember talking to her about the parts of cooking she enjoyed. What I do remember talking to her about was diets—mine and hers. By my mid-teens and early twenties, both of us were dieting and constantly scolding ourselves. She once told *People* magazine, "Valerie could probably work on watching her weight a little more." I was twenty-six and probably weighed 126 pounds. Sigh.

I'm sure she was talking to herself through me. But by sending me these recipes, she was, in her own motherly way, resetting the conversation. I was fifty-two, and she was seventy-five. It was about time we unpacked this passion that both of us shared and used it as a bridge to communicate in a new way. At the same time, I was starting a new conversation with myself about my life. I wasn't aware that it ran that deep. I didn't know a new door had been opened. I merely thought I was working on a cookbook.

But I discovered that it was so much more. First, I had to reconcile the fact that I was the most famous dieter in the whole United States, a spokesperson and role model for dieters who was authoring a cookbook that had nothing to do with being on a diet. I was upfront with my readers. *This is not a diet book.* It was a message to myself and the world. A coming out of sorts. I was coming out of the pantry. I wasn't declaring myself fat or thin as I had on umpteen TV commercials the past three years. I was declaring myself free.

*This book is about appreciating, celebrating, and enjoying good food—and not being afraid to eat it.*

If only it had been that easy. I went through the process of selecting recipes, making them, eliminating those that I thought fell short of the experience I wanted to share, adding new recipes, curating a balance and flow, and working with professional testers and editors to ensure that readers could follow the recipes and get the same results.

By the end, I loved the book and was proud of myself. There was just one problem. While I was promoting it on talk shows, I felt like a fake. I had so many doubts and questions. Why was I doing this? Was I a real cook? Was I confusing my fans and followers? Was I being authentic to myself? Or better still, after losing so much weight, had I found a new way to use food to torture myself? Why had I even written a cookbook?

As I said, I had started a new conversation with myself. I had to figure out what I was hearing.

. . . . . . . . .

I found myself asking more and deeper questions: How do we know who we are? How do we know who we are supposed to be?

I knew I was Valerie, the third of five children born to Nancy and Andrew (Andy) Bertinelli. I knew I was a mother. I knew I had been married and divorced and had recently remarried. I knew I had lost fifty pounds, gained some back, and run the Boston Marathon. I knew I got lucky at age fifteen when Norman Lear cast me in *One Day at a Time*, where I spent nine seasons and literally grew up in front of America. I knew I liked old Elton John songs, cats, and crossword puzzles. And I knew I was still riding a wave of luck by getting to work with an incredible group of smart, funny, talented, and beautiful women—Betty White, Wendie Malick, and Jane Leeves—on the series *Hot in Cleveland.*

But was I supposed to be acting—or still acting? A better question was this: Was acting all I was supposed to be doing? Or was moving into the kitchen the next step? How was I supposed to know? Or was not knowing part of the deal? Was that the point— to try, learn, grow, and see what happened? This was the dialogue I was having with myself, and writing the cookbook only amplified it. I was reminded of listening to one of Ed's new songs in the old 5150 studio. He turned the music up loud, then *louder*, until there was no escape. The sound consumed you.

Was it good? Would people like it? None of that mattered as long as Ed liked it.

I told my manager that I had an idea for another cookbook. I would go to Italy, explore my family's roots, cook there, and bring back recipes.

"Great," he said. "Let's also pitch it as a TV series called *Valerie Goes to Italy and All She Got Were Recipes for a Cookbook.*"

We took it to the Food Network, where they said the idea was too travel oriented. Then we pitched it to the Travel Channel, whose executives said it was too food focused for them and suggested that we take it to the Food Network. In the meantime, the Food Network called me back in and said they liked me and offered me an ITK.

"What's an ITK?" I asked.

An *in the kitchen* show, they explained. Like Rachael Ray's.

I lit up. Rachael was one of my heroes. I had guested on her show several times while promoting my first cookbook. In person, she was exactly as she seemed on TV: the friendliest, the smartest, and the hardest worker. I occasionally made her thirty-minute meals while watching her show. The biggest thing I learned from her was to let some things go and keep moving forward—good advice that could be applied to anything.

At that point, I found myself stepping into a brand-new role—as myself. I had traded a script for a skillet, and while I wasn't altogether unfamiliar with pots and pans, and slicing and dicing, cooking in front of cameras presented challenges. It was nerve-wracking. It was hard. It had the potential to embarrass me. And everything had to be done looking up at the cameras, not down at the food. If you're Ina Garten or Bobby Flay, that's as easy as riding a bike one-handed. But I was Valerie from Studio City. My cooking experience ranged from fixing my son's dinners to hosting my book club. I had a lot to learn.

That was the fun part. In May 2015, the week after shooting ended on *Hot in Cleveland*, I was practicing recipes in the Food Network test kitchens in Manhattan. The kitchens occupied a large floor atop the bustling Chelsea Market. My culinary producer, Mary Beth Bray, welcomed me with my own crisp, white, double-breasted chef's coat. It was personalized with my name stitched in blue cursive. It was a lovely gesture, but in no way did I think of myself as a chef, not then and not now all these years later. I was a cook learning how to cook.

The kitchens were crowded with multiple counters, stoves, ranges, refrigerators, and shelves of ingredients. I was there for a week and saw numerous people come in and out to work and experiment, including Alex Guarnaschelli. She was shooting *Chopped* right next door, and being a fan, I was thrilled to meet her.

Aside from the occasional star chef sighting, though, the people working in the kitchen were highly trained chefs who worked behind-the-scenes concocting and testing recipes for various shows and the Food Network's magazine. They were impressive to watch. Their movements were full of practiced intention and efficiency. Periodically, I heard someone shout the warnings you hear in a professional kitchen: "Watch it," "Behind you," "Hot," "Coming through."

Being there was exciting, intimidating, and pretty dang awesome. I felt the thrill of being in a place where I was going to learn and grow my repertoire, not only as a cook but as a fifty-something woman whose soul was ready to be nourished. I trusted the show's executive producer, Ronnie Weinstock, to not let me fail, and I worked closely with Mary Beth, an unflappable young woman with a baby-faced smile that reminded me of Renée Zellweger's. Inspired by Julia Child, Mary Beth had studied in Paris but had worked in several different fields before giving in to her passion for food. In that regard, we were on the same path.

We were similar in another way, too. When I asked what she liked to do away from work, she laughed, and said, "It's all about food—thinking about it, tasting, and doing research." I thought about food, too, but in a more complicated sense. Seeing that I was super nervous, then hearing me admit that I was really afraid of messing up, she gave my arm a reassuring squeeze, and said, "You can do it."

Hearing that, from her, was the tiny push I needed. We started cooking recipes from my cookbook, and it was pure fun and joy. Mary Beth had researched all of them and had recommendations for streamlining them or adding things to update them and bring out more flavor since a number of them had come from my mother and grandmother. On the second day, I couldn't wait to get back in the kitchen. By day three, I felt at home there.

Actually, it was better than home. People were cutting things for me and whisking away dirty bowls and dishes to get cleaned. Unlike acting, the gratification was nearly instantaneous. After twenty to forty minutes of work, there was usually something delicious to taste. Nobody ever ordered lunch. Those working in the kitchens put everything they made on a back counter for everyone to taste, enjoy, and comment on. Every day I put my dishes out. Out of the corner of my eye, I watched to see who tried some and whether they seemed to like it. Finally, at the end of the week, the day came when I got the reaction that every cook wants.

I set out my Sicilian love cake. It was chocolate, the same traditional version I made at home, where the cake was famous for appearing on birthdays and special occasions. It's typically made with a marble cake mix, ricotta, mascarpone, and chocolate pudding. My version is a rich chocolate devil's food cake mix with ricotta, chocolate pudding, and a little extra mascarpone. I forgot that I was in the Food Network kitchen. I could have been back at home. It felt natural and right and okay for me to share my excitement.

"Oh my God," I said, as I spooned the entire container of ricotta into a bowl, then added the mascarpone. "I just got a whiff of this and the chocolate cake batter that's already in the pan, and I think I might be in heaven."

Mary Beth smiled. "Spoken like a true cook."

"But it's not fancy," I said, suddenly doubting myself.

"That's not the goal—or the requirement," she counseled.

After fifty minutes, we took it out of the oven and let it cool. After applying the frosting, I dipped my finger in the bowl and declared the whole thing picture-perfect.

However, as with TV shows and movies, the final word wasn't up to me. The critics checked in midway through lunch when one of the chefs tasted the last piece and asked who made the chocolate cake. A small chorus of voices chimed in: "Yeah, who made that cake?" Rather modestly, I raised my hand. "It's amazing," someone said. A handful of people applauded, which made me very happy.

I smiled at Mary Beth, who nodded approvingly, and then I did something that I was well-practiced in: I took a bow.

. . . . . . . . .

Still, being around so many amazing chefs was a role that caused me to continually question whether I belonged, and I had to prove to myself that I did. Ratings was one barometer, and the reception to season one of *Valerie's Home Cooking* showed that I easily passed that test. Fans praised the show for being real and making meals that looked like the meals they made. Respect from my fellow Food Network hosts was another measure, and I couldn't have received more support from the gang. The same was true of my family and friends.

Only one person sounded a shrill note of criticism and doubt, and I had a helluva time convincing her to keep quiet. Even though I was the only one who heard her, that was enough. After years of telling people what they could and couldn't eat to lose weight and stay slim, I felt like a fraud showing them how to make lasagna, quick bread, gumbo, and my Neapolitan holiday cookies for chrissakes. I had an even harder time connecting with what I was doing and saying in front of the camera.

That conversation—the one in my head—was harder to change. When you're on a diet—and when you have dieted most of your life—you have trained yourself not to have a relationship with food, not to genuinely sit down and eat with other people, not to have relationships during mealtime, and not to relate to food in any way other than seeing it as bad. All of a sudden, I had to show up. The way I had done in Italy.

I had to reframe my relationship to food and myself in a way where success was based on the way I felt about myself rather than the same old numbers on the scale, and that was something that didn't happen overnight.

But help came from someone unexpected: my great-grandmother. Just before I pitched my show to the Food Network, I went on the TLC series *Who Do You Think You Are?* and received a report on my family's genealogy. I traveled to England to research my mother's side and to Italy to learn about my father's side. It turned out that my mother was related to a prominent family of Quakers named Claypoole, whose lineage could be traced to King Edward I. Dozens of other distant relatives—names in thick, dusty books in London's College of Arms—filled in the blanks.

My father's side was more pertinent to the moment. My father had an old scratched black-and-white photograph of my grandmother, then a young girl, and several grown women standing by a gelato cart in Lanzo Torinese, Italy. He wasn't able to identify the other women. This was an excellent starting point for the investigation, and it turned out that the woman behind the cart was my great-grandmother, Maria Francesca Possio Crosa. It was thanks to her, I was to learn, that cooking was in my blood.

When I got to Lanzo, I found out that Maria had worked as a cook at a home in San Remo. There she fell in love with the maintenance man, Francesco Crosa. They had two children, a girl, Angelina—my Nonnie—and a boy, Giorgio. Despite their jobs, they were still on the poverty list for nearly twenty years. To make extra money, my great-grandmother sold her homemade gelato. After Francesco died suddenly of a heart attack, she used her gelato savings to buy tickets to the United States for herself and her children.

It was 1915, and she was tired of being poor. She thought she would have a better life in America. She settled in Lackawanna County, Pennsylvania, and married an Italian man named Gregorio Mancia. I grew up hearing that he was shot dead during a poker game. In reality, he attempted to shoot my great-grandmother, who dodged the bullet and played dead. Thinking he had killed her, Gregorio went into the bedroom and shot himself. After that, my great-grandmother was finished with men. I don't blame her.

Her daughter—my Nonnie—grew up and met Nazzareno

Bertinelli, another character. He had left a wife and a three-year-old boy in Italy to come to America. I don't know if my Nonnie knew that about him. My brothers and I certainly didn't until many years later. My Nonnie and Nazzareno married and had three children, my father and my Aunts Adeline and Norma. Nonnie's handmade pasta was what I remembered most about her from my childhood — that and her and my aunts teaching my mother how to make gnocchi, risotto, polenta and sausages, and fresh bread.

Most weekends we had a family dinner at my Aunt Adeline's house, and my grandmother was in the basement kitchen with my aunts and my mother, cooking and telling stories. I remember gallon jugs of red wine on the long table in the middle of the room and the smell of butter, olive oil, garlic, fresh herbs, and baking bread — everything that smells delicious in a kitchen.

To me, family was always one of the many wonderful and essential ingredients that went into cooking. I remember the laughter and talking and affection at the table as people ate, and also the way everyone anticipated the meal as the rich aromas filtered through the house. But above all else, I remember the way the women responsible for making the meal were hugged and complimented and showered with love.

It was this legacy that food had among the women in my family that gave me the encouragement I needed to embrace this passion of mine, this new and maybe next chapter in my life. It was calling me and I was listening. This was part of who I was and who I was supposed to be. It wasn't about beating Bobby Flay or trying to outdo Giada. It wasn't about pretending I was a great chef or knew more than I did. It was about giving myself permission to connect to my heritage and enjoy food and everything associated with it.

It was about being me. And like my mom's recipe for lasagna, that was something I returned to again and again.

# Sicilian Chocolate Love Cake

Sometimes all you need is love . . . love cake, that is.

| | | | |
|---|---|---|---|
| 1 | box chocolate cake mix, plus the ingredients called for in its directions | | Canola oil, for preparing the pan |

## Mascarpone-Ricotta Filling

| | | | |
|---|---|---|---|
| 28 | ounces ricotta cheese (3½ cups) | 3 | large eggs |
| 4 | ounces mascarpone (½ cup) | ¾ | cup sugar |
| | | ⅛ | teaspoon kosher salt |

## Cocoa-Mascarpone Frosting

| | | | |
|---|---|---|---|
| 10 | ounces mascarpone (1¼ cups) | 1 | 3.9-ounce box instant chocolate pudding mix |
| 1 | cup whole milk | 1 | tablespoon sugar |

Preheat the oven according to the cake mix directions. Coat a 9-by-13-inch pan with canola oil. Prepare the cake batter according to the cake mix directions, pour into the prepared pan, and set aside.

To make the filling: Combine the ricotta, mascarpone, eggs, sugar, and salt in the bowl of a stand mixer and whisk until smooth. Gently pour the filling onto the cake pan of chocolate batter so the top is completely white. Bake until a skewer inserted in the center comes out clean and the chocolate layer has risen to the top, about 40 minutes. Let the cake cool completely.

To make the frosting: Just before serving, blend together the mascarpone, milk, chocolate pudding mix, and sugar in the bowl of a stand mixer until smooth. Using an offset spatula, spread the frosting evenly over the cake and serve.

# The Way Leon Looks at Me

## DECEMBER 2019

WHILE ED RESTS IN his hospital bed, recovering from the effects of a treatment, I am having a conversation with his assistant, Leon. Leon is a sharp, sophisticated young man whom Ed met in Germany during one of his trips there for cancer treatment. After starting as Ed's chef, Leon has become more like a twenty-four-hour nurse-slash-caregiver, driving him to appointments when Wolfie is busy, making sure he stays on top of his medications, preparing his meals, and ensuring that Ed has what he wants. They get along great, and I understand why.

It's my first one-on-one, in-depth conversation with Leon. He speaks four languages and has traveled extensively. He tells me about the meals he likes preparing for Ed. I share my stories about cooking for Ed when we were married and how I learned to make his favorite dishes from Mrs. Van Halen.

After gushing about my trip to Italy where I fell in love with food all over again and hearing about Leon's gustatory excursions there, I tell him about my Nonnie and Aunt Adeline's cappelletti, because I can't talk about Italy or my love of cooking without referencing them, and soon Leon and I are discussing recipes, ingredients, and techniques with such passion that I almost forget we are in a hospital room with Ed.

"Edward told me that you have a cooking show on television," Leon says.

"Yes, I have a lot of fun on it," I say.

"It's so great that you love food," he says.

I chuckle. "Well, look at me."

Leon stares at me, confused. He doesn't get it. My attempt to use a self-deprecating quip to infer that I am fat does not register with him. He does not see me the way I see myself, which is heavy, struggling, not my best self, and not who I want to be. I wish it were different. I want to look at me the way Leon looks at me. He doesn't see the fat. He just sees my knowledge and enthusiasm. *Why can't I do that?*

Seriously. Why can't I?

I get in my car and drive home fixated on this question. Since my teens, I have struggled with body image. The person I see in the mirror is fat, flawed, and in need of fixing. No one else has seen me that way. Ed adored me at any size (and once, during our heaviest days of partying, he actually told me that I was too thin). And Tom asked me out on our first date when my weight was at an all-time high. I have always been the dissenter. Even after running the Boston Marathon a few days before my fiftieth birthday and finishing in five hours and fifteen minutes, I stared at a picture of myself crossing the finish line, exhausted and elated, and thought, *Oh my God, my thighs look so big.*

Now, a decade later, I have lost both of my parents and my son's father is fighting cancer and the last thing I need is to hate myself because of some number on the scale.

As I keep telling myself—and the whole world—*Enough already.*

Morning comes and I have a come-to-Jesus moment with myself. Instead of stepping on the scale as I always do, I stand in front of the bathroom mirror, and say, "Can I just at least not hate myself today? Can I at least do that? Can I not chastise myself because my jeans are a little tight? Can I get out of bed and look at the beautiful sunrise, appreciate the beauty surrounding me, enjoy hearing my cats purr, watching Luna's tail wag, and feel gratitude for the life that I've been given? Can I just love myself today?"

I do not know if this is a surrender or a declaration of war.

It feels like both.

A few days later, I have a similar, less strident conversation with myself. Maybe I don't have to struggle so much. Maybe I can just love myself today and see what happens.

I like that idea.

What exactly is it that I am trying to fix? What's broken?

At my age, I should no longer be holding my body to the same standard I did when I was eighteen, thirty, or even forty; though at this point, I am not even sure what that standard is or whether there should be a standard other than healthy and loved. All I have ever told myself is that I need to change. It started in elementary school when a teacher pointed to my stomach, and said, "You better watch that." At thirteen, I got it in my head that I had big hips, what I referred to as child-bearing hips, and I began to see myself as too curvy.

Two years later, I was on the set of *One Day at a Time* and comparing myself to my costar Mackenzie Phillips, who was tall and thin and beautiful. I thought she had the perfect figure, like the sixties supermodel Twiggy. She was everything I wasn't. During an interview at the time, I actually told a reporter that I had a "very serious weight problem" and looked "like a tub of lard" when I stood next to Mackenzie.

I was fifteen or sixteen years old then. I thought I had an hourglass shape and I was embarrassed by it. I always wanted to be something other than what I was: taller, blonder, thinner. Every morning I got on the scale, and the rest of the day was an effort to make up for the number I saw. I never thought about enjoying meals. I told myself to be good. At the end of the day, I was either bad or I cheated or I slipped.

On the set, I hated going into wardrobe for fittings. I wanted to die whenever they said that they had to get a bigger size for me. I didn't realize that they were bringing in small sizes because they thought of me as tiny and that the next sizes they got for me were still smalls. I thought the smaller the number on the scale, the more beautiful I was and the more jobs I would get. But it didn't work that way. I went up for the movie *Footloose*, and when the part went to Lori Singer, I assumed that it was because I wasn't as skinny or as beautiful as she was.

The same thing happened with the movie *Cocoon*, and I was devastated. I assumed that the people doing the casting thought I was ugly and fat or that something else was wrong with me. It never occurred to me that I might not have been a good enough actor or that I didn't match what they had in mind. I just didn't get it.

· · · · · · · · ·

At forty-seven years old, I signed up to be a spokesperson for Jenny Craig. I was public about my reasons. I announced to the world that I was fat—my weight was at an all-time high—and the goal I set for myself was to get thin. Finally. That was so me. I set up an all-or-nothing situation where the stakes were not only disappointment but also public shame and humiliation if I didn't reach my goal, to say nothing of the devastation that this would cause privately.

The plan was reflective of my mindset at the time—broken,

skewed, and unrealistic. I wasn't trying to get healthy or deal with the reasons I had gained weight over the years—the currents of unhappiness, sadness, and discontent that flowed beneath my public cheer. I wanted to get thin. The two are not the same.

But it also showed my determination to survive. I had split from Ed in May of 2002 and I refused to take money from him. As a single working mom, I needed to make money. I wasn't getting work as an actress. Jenny Craig was a good job, and it was going to make me thin. It was the best of the two worlds that mattered to me, and I put everything I had into making sure I succeeded.

The deal called for me to lose thirty pounds in eight months. I did it in three. My manager, Marc Schwartz, negotiated a new deal for ten more pounds. After I lost those next ten pounds faster than expected, they asked if I would consider fifty pounds and pose in a bikini for the cover of *People* magazine. I agreed under two conditions: First, that we avoid mention of the fifty pounds because I already knew it was impossible to maintain that weight loss; and second, that I wasn't going to try to get into said bikini until ten days before the scheduled photo shoot.

That whole time I followed Jenny Craig's program as if I were a nun who had taken a vow of celibacy, which was the way it felt at times. I ate preprepared meals, worked out, talked with my sponsor, and stepped on the scale for my weekly weigh-ins. The numbers kept going down. I was exhausted. I told myself that I was in training. I was going to get skinny. I was finally going to have the body I always wanted.

The bikini photo shoot was scheduled for the end of March 2009. Ten days before, my manager called me in the morning.

"How are you feeling?" he asked.

"Let's do it," I said.

For the next week and a half, I barely ate. I wanted to get in that bikini and see abs and definition, and I did. The photo shoot was done in total secrecy. No one on the crew was allowed to bring their phone onto the set. A week later, I was on the cover of *People* magazine wearing a tiny green bikini (which, by the way, was a large—even at my smallest, one hundred and twenty-two pounds, I still wore a large, evidence of how screwed-up the fashion industry is with sizing). A Jenny Craig commercial also ran nonstop.

"Now nothing's stopping me from diving into summer," I said, as I did a back dive into a swimming pool.

My smile was real. The splash was real. I was ecstatic. I proved that I could do something really hard if I put my mind to it—and I was thin.

I was happy that day although I almost fainted on the set. That night, I drank champagne. I enjoyed putting on my jeans without lying on the bed to pull up the zipper and slipping into a dress without having to pull two or three roomier alternatives out of my closet. But that feeling didn't last much longer than those champagne bubbles. Neither did the weight loss. I started gaining as soon as the photo shoot ended. That was just one of many realities. Whether I was a size two, an eight, or a fourteen, I was still me.

That was never more apparent than when I started working with Wendie Malick and Jane Leeves on *Hot in Cleveland*. Both women were tall, skinny, beautiful, and gorgeous, and I thought, *Here I am again, the one with the hourglass figure, short and round.* All my insecurities came out as if Jenny Craig had never happened.

I remember one day at the end of the second season when we were preparing for a scene where Wendie, Jane, and I had to wear the same little black dress for Elka's wedding. After getting dressed, I stood in the wardrobe room trying not to cry. I had seen the two other women looking tall and skinny and stunning, and there I was, short, fat, and round.

"Do I have to wear the same dress as them?" I asked our costume designer, Lori Eskowitz-Carter. "Couldn't I wear one that's not so tight?"

She was pained by my pain.

"Valerie, you are beautiful," she said. "Why do you do this to yourself?"

"Thank you, but stop it," I said, unable to handle the compliment and eager to get out from in front of the mirror.

"Why don't you believe that you are beautiful?"

. . . . . . . . .

It's the stories we tell ourselves. In the early 2000s, I heard about a study conducted by a Japanese researcher who studied water samples exposed to positive and negative messages. The water that was praised and thanked and loved looked clean and clear under a microscope. The water that was criticized and told that it was hated lost its purity and developed an unpleasant toxicity when studied under a microscope.

Whether these studies stand up to scientific scrutiny is debatable, but in a practical way, they make perfect sense to me. If you start every day by getting on a scale and telling yourself that you failed, you will feel like a failure. If you begin every meal by telling yourself not to eat because the food is bad for you and will screw up the number on the scale, you will approach every meal as if it's something to fear rather than enjoy. Food is not the enemy.

I have always believed my poor body image began in elementary school when my teacher made that damaging comment about my tummy. I don't know if I was even aware of my body before he said that. But that was only the most obvious source of confusion and insecurity. I think the root causes may have started earlier. While my mother was pregnant with me, my older brother, Mark, died after wandering unwatched into a friend's barn and drinking poison out of a soda bottle. He was seventeen months old.

I was born only a few months later. I was literally born into grief. My young parents were still trying to get through that horrendous experience. I believe that I absorbed their sense of loss and sadness like the water did in that experiment. My parents never hid this tragedy from me or my brothers, but they didn't talk about it, either. It was too painful for them. I didn't learn about it until I was in my early teens. Only after my Nonnie died and I went back to Delaware for the funeral did I finally see Mark's grave. The two were buried near each other.

I remember reading Mark's headstone while holding Wolfie in my arms. At the time, Wolfie was about the same age as Mark was when he died. I have always said that I couldn't imagine the pain my parents went through after losing their child. However, I could imagine it. And I did. I remember tightening my grip on Wolfie as tears washed down my face. It was the first time that I grieved for my brother, and I began to understand my parents a little better.

I have returned to that feeling many times over the years in an effort to process and understand the impact Mark's death had on all of us. I don't know how my parents dealt with it or each other. My father had the ability to put on a stoic mask and soldier on. But I don't think my mother ever allowed herself to really grieve. Once, when I was pregnant, she said, "If it's a boy, you're going to name him Mark, right?" Aside from that one time, we never talked about him or how my parents got through that terrible time.

No wonder, like me, she ended up on a lifelong diet because she ate her feelings instead of working to understand them. I know there was joy surrounding my arrival, but I wonder if more was expected from me.

I knew my parents' love for me was without question and that my birth had nothing to do with the tragedy of losing Mark. Still, before I was even born, there was a message sent to me that my role was to please others and bring enough happiness to fill a gaping hole, a task that could never be completed and that also missed the real point—much like the ten pounds I would always be trying to lose. I assumed a role that was never mine to fill. I never put it together until I allowed myself to do what my parents didn't know how to: take the space to grieve what wasn't, what isn't, and what can never be.

It took me until I was nearly sixty years old, but I finally understood that this feeling of trying to make up for my parents' loss was as impossible as finding happiness in a number on the scale. I have to consciously remind myself that it doesn't make sense, and in its place, I need to create a new, more rational, and healthier narrative.

· · · · · · · · ·

How do you change the narrative?

By being present and aware.

My body is perfectly fine. Why am I so critical of it? Why do I treat it like an emotional trash can?

*Enough already.*

Bodies are bodies—each one different and unique, even with people who are the same size and weight. They are neither good nor bad.

They can be healthy or unhealthy.

But it's what they contain that matters most—the head and the heart.

This body of mine functions properly and performs on command; and I suppose that if it could talk on its own it would ask, "Why do you hate me? I get you up in the morning. I make your coffee. I get you upstairs and downstairs. I take your dog for walks. I call your cats and answer the phone. I help you smell the roses. I know how to open a bottle of wine. I dance. I swim. I think. I laugh. I fight off germs. I inhale and exhale. I ran a marathon. I created a brand-new life. I taught that brand-new life how to drive (and freaked out only a few times). I'm here for you all the time."

I finally hear it and know what to say in response: "I don't hate you. I don't mean to treat you badly. I am sorry for the past. Thank you for everything you have done for me and continue to do. I am trying to change. I want to treat you better. I hope we are together and continue this relationship for a very long time. I love you."

When I begin to hear the old voices in my head now, I try to close my eyes and breathe through the moment. I calmly tell myself that I am kind, I am good, and I am beautiful just the way I am right now. At this age. In this body. Sometimes I choose other words. Sometimes the words don't register with me. Sometimes I have to get up and move. The important thing is to do something to change the narrative in my head. Our bodies are 70 percent water, I remind myself. Talk nicely.

Like this afternoon. When I start to have one of those moments where the anxiety creeps up on me, I get up and go for a walk in the backyard. I pick a few grapefruits from one of the trees. I also see oranges and lemons that are ready to be brought inside. And kumquats. My kumquat tree is a marvel that almost seems to be speaking to me. The fruit begins to ripen at the bottom, then fills out in the middle, and finally changes color at the top. I fill a small bucket with the bite-size fruit and bring it into the kitchen, thinking I'll make some kumquat liqueur. There's more: peaches, guavas, pomegranates. I catch myself smiling at this blessing of abundance.

I am also feeling inspired. I want to create something delicious for dinner tonight. Maybe a lemon pasta with shrimp. Maybe a dessert. Maybe both.

This is how I change the narrative.

. . . . . . . . .

My mom used to make a pineapple upside-down cake that was always one of my favorites. With the fruit I have picked, I am going to make a variation of that, my upside-down citrus cake. It's tangy, sweet, and refreshing. I melt butter and mix brown sugar and granulated white sugar. Once it turns into a buttery smooth caramel, I pour it into a pan. Then I layer in slices of my oranges and a grapefruit, and pour in some orange liqueur. I make cake batter, scoop it over the fruit and bake at 350 degrees for fifty to sixty minutes.

As it bakes, the cats and the dog find their way into the kitchen, and I know why. Something smells good and sweet and delicious. They give me a look that says, *You're driving us crazy again*. Once upon a time, I would have spent all this time telling myself why this upside-down citrus cake was bad for me and denying myself even the smallest taste until — guess what — I would have eaten a couple of pieces and hated myself the rest of the day.

But today I am reveling in the process, from gathering the fresh ingredients from my trees to the bakery scent that fills my kitchen. I can't wait to share it. Look at me: I love food. You can see why.

# Upside-Down Citrus Cake

Don't think about it—just do something nice for yourself. Making this cake is a step in the right direction. It's beautiful, refreshing, and sweet—everything I try to tell myself and you should tell yourself, too. You'll thank yourself later.

## Topping

4 tablespoons unsalted butter, plus more for the pan

1 small to medium grapefruit

1 navel orange

1 Cara Cara or blood orange

½ cup granulated sugar

¼ cup light brown sugar

1 tablespoon orange liqueur, optional

## Cake

1¾ cups all-purpose flour

1 teaspoon baking powder

½ teaspoon baking soda

½ teaspoon salt

1 stick (8 tablespoons) unsalted butter, softened

1 cup granulated sugar

2 large eggs

1 teaspoon pure vanilla extract

1 cup buttermilk

*(recipe continued on next page)*

*For the Topping*

Preheat the oven to 350 degrees F. Generously butter a 9-inch round cake pan and line the bottom with parchment paper.

Use a fine grater to zest 1 teaspoon of zest from the grapefruit, navel orange, and blood orange (for a total of 1 tablespoon zest). Reserve the zest for the cake.

Cut the top and bottom off of each citrus and place them with a flat side on the cutting board. Then, following the curve of the fruit, use a sharp knife to cut off the peels and as much of the white pith as possible. Slice the fruit crosswise into ¼-inch-thick rounds; carefully remove any seeds.

Combine the butter and both sugars in a small saucepan and warm over medium-low heat until melted. Pour into the prepared cake pan and spread evenly. Top with the citrus rounds so they fit very snugly and are slightly overlapping (you may not use every slice). Drizzle with the orange liqueur, if using.

*For the Cake*

Whisk the flour, baking powder, baking soda, and salt together in a medium bowl. Put the butter, sugar, and reserved zest in another bowl and beat with an electric mixer on medium-high speed until light and fluffy, about 3 minutes. Add the eggs one at a time, beating after each addition. Beat in the vanilla. Add the flour mixture in 3 batches, alternating with the buttermilk, beginning and ending with the flour; mix until just combined.

Pour the cake batter over the citrus and bake until a wooden pick inserted into the center comes out clean, 50 to 60 minutes. Run a sharp knife around the edge of the cake and let it cool for 15 minutes, then carefully invert it onto a platter, replacing any citrus that may have stuck to the pan. Serve slightly warm or at room temperature.

# Secret Ingredients

## APRIL 2020

O N MY SIXTIETH BIRTHDAY, I wake up at three-thirty in the morning to get ready for an appearance on the *Today* show. I wash my face, brush my hair, put on a business-appropriate blouse, and pour coffee in my eyes. Or it feels like I did. It is early on the West Coast. The show celebrated by sending me two rosemary plants, two lavender plants, and two huge bouquets of flowers—one gift for each decade. At a little past five in the morning, I am live on the air with Hoda, Savannah, and Carson. I uncork a bottle of my favorite champagne, which they also sent, and I share a virtual toast with everybody.

I laughingly say it is too early to drink, and at that hour, it does seem a little ridiculous, though, as we make jokes, I remember occasions when I was on the road with Ed and we rolled into our hotel room around this same time and had just one more. I wasn't always the goody two-shoes people imagined. In fact, once I am off the air, I say to myself, *What the hell, you're only sixty once in your life*, and I take a sip of champagne.

Woo-hoo. Wild times. Par-*tee*.

The girl's still got it.

And then the girl changes back into her T-shirt and sweats, and goes back to bed.

· · · · · · · · ·

I have no qualms about hitting this milestone. I have thought about it more and more with the approach of the actual date, April 23. Sixty definitely sounded older and more AARP-worthy than fifty-nine, which itself held a certain significance, like waiting in traffic to make a left-hand turn from one stage of life into another. I was more afraid of the way I was going to feel than the way I actually do feel throughout the day.

After I get up, I enjoy a leisurely day of doing nothing. I read the paper and sip more coffee. I make some of my favorite blueberry, banana, and oat muffins. I love muffins, especially these, and the delicious smell from the oven takes me back to my childhood, when my mom made blueberry muffins or banana bread and I hovered in the kitchen waiting for the first bite of those freshly baked, warm treats. I am ten years old again.

I use fresh blueberries and bananas, of course, but as I whip up this batch, the generous splash of vanilla the recipe calls for, while seemingly minor, stands out to me as a crucial ingredient, almost a secret ingredient that gives the muffins their flavor. Or if it is not entirely responsible for the flavor, it enhances the taste in the same way butter finishes off pasta sauce, lemon squeezed on top of a cantaloupe brings out the lush juices, and rosemary in vegetables somehow turns every bite into a celebration of the garden.

"There are no such things as secrets in the kitchen," wrote the late, great LA chef Michael Roberts, whose restaurant, Trumps, was an institution on a par with Spago in the eighties. "But there are secret ingredients, those ingredients that are not tasted but would be missed if they were omitted. A secret ingredient is one that mysteriously improves the flavor of a dish without calling attention to itself."

I treat my birthday the same way: by making sure I add the secret ingredients. I go for a walk. I smell the roses. I cut some flowers. Spring is in bloom. Wolfie comes by but stays outside in the backyard because of Covid-19. I meet him out there. It is weird and strange and sad, especially because I don't get a hug—not from him or anyone else. I field birthday texts from friends I might normally see on my birthday and tell myself to feel the love they are sending me.

At night, my closest girlfriends send over takeout from one of our favorite restaurants—the French bistro where we would have gathered were it not for the virus-inspired lockdown—and eat together over Zoom. It's not the same as in person, but we make the best of it, telling stories and laughing for a couple of hours. I didn't really hang out with girlfriends in my twenties, and I didn't really have any back then. I was always surrounded by guys—Ed and all of the techs, engineers, and musicians who worked with him at the studio and on tour. It was like the Scout troop from the dark side of the moon.

But tonight is one more instance of the way my girlfriends have helped me make new memories. We have held one another's hands through major and minor life events—health scares, birthdays, anniversaries, job changes, career decisions, elections, and now a pandemic. We bring so much shared history to the table—or to Zoom in this case—and the experience never disappoints.

I get insights and understanding I wouldn't otherwise have had, and for however long we are together—tonight it's for a couple of hours—I rarely think about myself, not in the brooding, judgmental way I do when I am alone. Instead, I am giving, sharing, serving—whether its food, an opinion, encouragement, support, advice, or laughter.

Remember poet Shel Silverstein's children's book *The Giving Tree*? It's about a tree that loved a little boy more than she loved herself. It ends with both of them having grown older, the boy an old man in need of a place to sit and rest and the tree now no more than a stump but still eager to help him in some way. "Come, Boy, sit down. Sit down and rest," she says. "And the boy did. And the tree was very happy."

This is at the core of my love of cooking. As I have redefined my relationship with food over the past decade—first with my trip to Italy, then by writing a cookbook, and then with the TV series—I have redefined my life and reconnected with values I consider important. My cooking is about a passion for the process: picking out ingredients, creating something new and delicious, then sharing it with other people.

When you are locked into a dieting mindset, you are not eating with other people. You are not able to have relationships during mealtime. You are distancing yourself from food, from other people, from yourself, and from life. Cooking enabled me to reconnect with everything I had denied myself and missed. It's a process that I work through daily, because old bad habits are slow to fade completely away, but I try, and try, and try, and when I am successful, like Shel Silverstein's giving tree, I am very happy.

· · · · · · · · ·

Someone asked what I want for my birthday. Here's what I want:

I want to be able to laugh like Julia Roberts, a kind of joyous, from-the-heart laugh that erupts from within and shakes the entire room.

I want my kid to be healthy and happy.

I want the same for my brothers and their wives and kids and my friends and their families.

I want people to have enough to eat and drink, especially kids.

I want there to be enough of whatever people need to pass around so everyone gets their fair portion.

That's it.

· · · · · · · · ·

You know what scares me about turning sixty? It's closer to eighty, and I think that's when I am going to die. I'll explain.

Many years ago, Ed and I went to a party at singer Sammy Hagar's house. At the time, he was living near us at the beach. There was a psychic at the party whom I had seen privately about a year earlier for help losing weight. At the time, I was one hundred and thirty-six pounds and thought I needed to lose ten pounds, which was a sure sign of crazy. But I was seeing a psychic for diet advice, so enough said.

The psychic started by asking what I had for breakfast. When I told him that I had an English muffin with peanut butter, he shuddered and backed away from me, as if hearing that had caused him to glimpse something horrific.

"No, no, no, no, Valerie," he scolded. "You can't do that. It sets you up wrong for the whole day."

I should have asked who was telling him that—was it his opinion or was someone on the other side providing this information, and if that was the case, who was it, because the women on my side of the family who might have been hovering around him would have said that this wasn't enough, and they would have encouraged me to eat even more. Nevertheless, I believed him. Breakfast became coffee, and I was thrilled when we crossed paths again at Sammy's.

We found a quiet place to sit and he gave me another reading. For whatever reason, this one focused on life and longevity. During the reading, he casually said that I was going to die in my early eighties and that Ed was going to pass away in his mid-sixties. Perhaps because he was so specific or perhaps because all of us wonder how long this inexplicable miracle of our existence is going to last, I never forgot what he said.

I recalled his reading after both of my parents passed, three years apart but at the same age of eighty-two. Ed, who had turned sixty-five in January, did not seem like he was about to walk through the exit door, but he wasn't having an easy time, either.

It made me think. If I had only twenty years left, what would I want to do? Why limit it to twenty years? What if I had only one day? Or one hour? What would I want to accomplish starting right now? The answer came to me in a flash. I want to stop wasting time. I want to love myself. I want to get off this treadmill of not loving myself. I want to be able to forgive myself for the slips and the tears and the moments when I don't feel strong or loving or kind. I want to be able to recognize and embrace life's delights when they appear. I want to give myself permission to always be me, whatever that looks and feels like at this age.

The best part of turning sixty is that I can say, "Enough already," and mean it. The number isn't important anymore. It's the feeling that is important. How do I feel? How am I making others feel? I spent a lifetime being told to step outside my comfort zone. I never want to leave it now. I want to spend the rest of my life the way author Anne Lamott described in her book *Plan B: Further Thoughts on Faith:* "Age has given me what I've been looking for my entire life—it's given me *me*. It has provided time and experience and failures and triumphs and time-tested friends who have helped me step into the shape that was waiting for me. I fit into me now." And you know what? That is exactly the size I want to feel comfortable in — me.

. . . . . . . . .

The question is, how do you do this? I spout all these things about wanting to be kinder and more loving to myself, as do so many other people, as if it's possible to flip a switch and be that person in seven steps. It is not. What I have found since saying, "Enough already," a few months ago is that it requires work. Every single day I have to remind myself that the way I want to love myself and experience joy is not so much an end goal as it is a value and an intention to realign with over and over again.

What I am learning and relearning and constantly reminding myself of is that joy, happiness, gratitude — all those things we all want, including love — won't find me. I have to go out and find them. All of us do. It works that way for everyone.

The good news is that instead of seven steps or fifteen steps or a whole how-to book there is only one step to being kinder and more loving: you follow your heart.

You just do it.

You follow your heart.

When you let it, your heart is always going to lead to the same place, a place of helping, giving, and being kind. I do this with food. I love to feed people. It fills my heart. I wish I had pushed myself in this direction ages ago — off the scale and away from the mirror to feeding others. I didn't know better. But the experience never fails to return the kindness and love I want to feel myself. It lets me see the me I like. It's the me that I never try to fix — because part of me doesn't feel like it needs fixing. It's kind and loving and proof that the most important part of me—my heart—is not broken.

By my birthday, I have been on lockdown for a month and a half. I hate what Covid has done to us. Everyone I know is confused, scared, pissed off, looking for answers, and grasping for hope. I want to invite them over and cook for them.

# No Time Like Today

## MAY 2020

I HAVE SOME ADVICE FOR anyone who has the urge to get in touch with someone important in their life, be it a parent, an aunt or uncle, your ex, a friend from the past, a former neighbor or teammate, a teacher or colleague: Do it. Listen to your gut and make the call, send the email, or write the DM. There is no time like today.

Your head is not always rational, but your heart is never wrong.

I say this because I am having trouble getting together with Ed. I am frustrated. It shouldn't be that difficult for us to see each other since we are in regular communication and frequently check in with each other via text. It started last November when I was in New York promoting *Valerie's Home Cooking*. While shopping at the Nintendo store, I FaceTimed with Wolfie to show him all the cool Zelda stuff they had, and on the way outside, I saw the big tree at Rockefeller Center and that made me think of Ed.

I call him and he picks up. I tell him where I am and that I am walking around Midtown Manhattan by myself. The last time the three of us were together in New York was on Van Halen's 2015 tour. We didn't spend a lot of time together, but we had fun, and Ed and I reminisce about it even though there isn't a lot to say.

"I just wanted you to know I was thinking about you," I say.

"Thanks. Have a good time there for me."

"I will. Love you."

"Love you, too."

Over the next few months, we want to get together but can't seem to make it work other than when Ed is in the hospital in January. Then I start work on my show, Covid hits, and I am too concerned about bringing the virus into his house and getting him sick even though I repeatedly test negative through the spring. We still text. Mostly mundane stuff. "So what shows are you watching?" he asks one day. I send him a few titles. "Thanks Val. ♥" Or else I just check in, no response necessary. "Thinking of you. Hope you're having a good day."

Ed and I split twenty years ago. People are always surprised at how close we have remained. I too sometimes marvel at the affection we still have for each other considering how much we hurt each other years ago. But we grew up and grew past our problems, and parenthood and the love we have always had for each other proved to be stronger and more resilient than anything else. We chose to remain friends and family—and worked at it.

Therapy got us through rough patches, but we always knew we didn't want to go through life without each other. That included second marriages. When Ed tied the knot with publicist Janie Liszewski in 2009, I sat on the groom's side. At my wedding to Tom the next year, Ed and Janie were there to toast our I dos. Ironically, both of our marriages are now unraveling. I haven't told him about Tom and me, and while Ed mentioned that his was likely headed for divorce, I wasn't comfortable pressing him for details. If I had been more inquisitive, I would have gone to his place more frequently these past few months to drop off meals, watch TV, or simply to keep him company.

It pains me to think he might have been alone or lonely. In the meantime, I couldn't get past whether bringing him pasta or watching a football game with him would be inappropriate. Now, I think, *Really Val? How is calling to ask "How ya doin'?" or "Are you hungry? Can I make you something?" inappropriate?* I should have learned my lesson that afternoon in 2018 when Ed and I crossed paths at the studio where Wolfie was rehearsing with his band. I was already there when Ed arrived. He gave me a kiss hello and sat down on a nearby sofa. My heart told me to get up and sit down next to him and put my arm around him, so we could be proud parents together.

*Just go do it,* I told myself.

But I didn't budge. Not right away. I was hesitant about overstepping boundaries even if I was the only one who saw them. One could say it was a case of me getting in my own way . . . again. Eventually I did move closer to him, and I was glad I did. Not only did Ed appreciate the company, but also when I asked how he was doing, he had news to share: he said that his cancer had spread to his brain. I stared at him, shocked, feeling myself go numb.

*What?*

"Yeah," he said, looking down at the floor, as if he couldn't believe what a huge bummer had been handed to him yet again.

He went on to explain that he had wrecked his motorcycle on Mulholland Drive and that the subsequent examination had turned up the results. As he shared the details, I noticed that I had draped my arm over his knees. It was something I had done automatically, without any thought, as a way of being close, though when I did notice, I immediately thought, *Uh-oh, this is kind of intimate.* It was kind of intimate—and perfectly appropriate for the situation.

So was the way I wrapped my arms around him and squeezed as hard as I could, trying to express everything that was so hard at that point: love, strength, and hope.

· · · · · · · · ·

My notions about what was appropriate were stupid. There is nothing wrong with letting someone know that you love them. Period.

I was thankful that Ed and I had our moment a year later in George Lopez's car on Thanksgiving, and I was a little more relaxed about seeing him after that, though I still missed opportunities for us to be together. One text exchange is particularly painful. We were going to get together for Thursday night football. I was going to fix us dinner. But that morning I got a text from Ed suggesting that we postpone.

"Let me go through today's radiation treatment first because I don't know how I'm going to feel afterward," he wrote. "Usually it's pretty shitty."

I understood, wished him well, and told him that I hadn't shopped for any ingredients yet so we could reschedule whenever he was up to it.

Late that afternoon, Ed texted me back to say that the machine had broken down and that he wasn't able to get the treatment so I could come over to watch the game. Because it was late and I was focused on bringing over dinner but hadn't gone to the store, I suggested picking another date. I wish I hadn't made seeing him contingent on dinner and had gone over there and just hung out for an hour. In reality, neither of us cared about dinner as much as we did about the time together. Like so many people, we weren't able to express it clearly.

Since then, he has continued to provide openings to hang out.

He has told me that he's getting back into football. He has asked what shows I am watching. But for some reason, I keep creating roadblocks, worrying about giving the wrong impression, then beating myself up afterward for overthinking things and ultimately wasting precious time we could spend together.

Story of my life. I turned down job interviews because I didn't want people to see me at a weight that I considered heavy. I stayed in my bedroom for days and weeks because I thought I was fat. I turned down dinner invitations with friends because I was *trying to be good*. And I wonder why I am crying out for joy and happiness?

How much time did I waste dieting in an effort to lose ten pounds? Time is something we have no business treating as if it were available in an unlimited supply and will always be there, like a half-used jar of pickle relish on a refrigerator shelf. For me, the waste has always come down to those ten pounds. Losing ten pounds was going to make me happy, prettier, content, finished. It consumed my life. Sometimes it still does. But when I look back at pictures of myself at fifty, at forty, at sixteen — at any age, really — I say to myself, *What were you thinking? What a waste of time.*

And the problem was never those ten pounds.

· · · · · · · · ·

So what do those ten pounds really represent?

Even when I lost those ten pounds, I didn't treat myself any better. The ten pounds weren't enough. Which begs the question: What will be enough? How about five hundred pounds? Don't laugh. Everybody who has measured happiness on a scale should think about this: I've been trying to lose ten pounds for forty-some years. I've lost and I've gained. Sometimes more, sometimes less. At a minimum, though, that adds up to four hundred pounds, and that hasn't been enough, which is absurd. It's like a dog chasing its tail. There is no end goal. It's just a dizzying, exhausting, endless circle.

Because it has never been about the weight. Each time I have talked about wanting or needing to lose those ten pounds, they have represented something else going on in my life, something that's making me sad, causing me pain, or making me anxious. When I was a teenager, it may have been a party I hoped to get invited to or a school test I wanted to ace. Later, I might have been stressing about something at work—clothes I wanted to wear, a part I wanted to get. When I was married to Ed, it was my anger and insecurity. After losing both of my parents within a three-year span, I gained weight, and instead of addressing my grief and sadness, I focused on the food I was eating and all that I said I couldn't eat.

And now it's Ed's health.

It's the concern I have for my son.

It's my own fear of losing someone whose life has been so integral to mine that I can't imagine being without him.

When I ask myself why I can't lose weight, what I'm really asking is why can't I get a grip. Why am I not dealing with what's really bothering me? Instead, the focus always goes to those ten pounds because that number and the weight itself is something I can target and seemingly control through willpower. If I can change the way I eat, I will lose weight. And if I lose weight, I will feel better. I will be able to get rid of the problem or problems that I'm not actually solving.

But that approach is backward. When you think about how the emotions, stress, worries, and anxieties that we carry around with us can feel like weight, you begin not only to understand what those ten pounds really mean, you can also actually feel them. Losing weight is a way of seeming to manage and control things that seem otherwise unmanageable and uncontrollable. But it doesn't work. I can't begin to recall how many times I have told myself that I will feel better about everything if I just lose those ten pounds. It seems so tangible, so doable, so easy. It's just ten pounds. Who can't lose ten pounds?

My hand is up.

Here's the problem. Trying to lose ten pounds or any other number of pounds does not address the real problems, and there is always something else, some other problem, and therefore there are another ten pounds that you or I decide we need to lose. Dieting may help us fit into a smaller pair of jeans, but it won't help us fit into our life. Trust me. Look at me. I know what I am talking about.

The goal is to live in the moment, not on the scale. Remind yourself that it's not the weight and that it never has been the weight. It's not those ten pounds. It's the problems that are attached to those ten pounds. When I look in the mirror these days, I see someone who is a little heavy, but what I really see is pain and sadness that I haven't dealt with. I can't diet those away. I have to work through them, and as I do, I believe there's a great possibility that the weight will follow.

I tell myself to take a deep breath. Muster the courage to confront the real issues, the pain, the grief, the sadness, the regrets, the fear. Talk about them. Allow yourself to cry. Forgive yourself for any mistakes you have made. Then, do your best to move through them and forward, knowing that this is the only way you will get to a better, healthier, and happier place.

And don't put it off. The time is today.

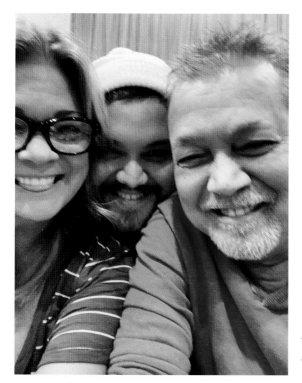

The spinach and crab dip night.

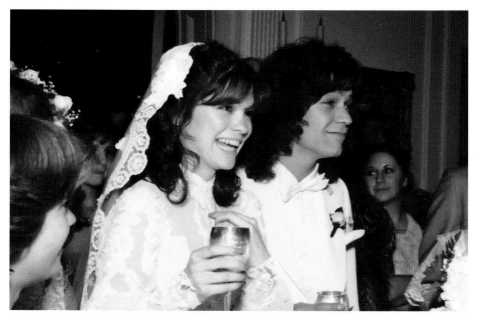

Enjoying our wedding day. Ed was twenty-six, but I wasn't old enough to legally drink yet. Don't tell anyone.

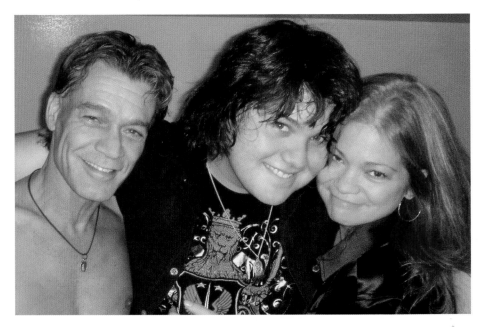

This is the first year Wolfie played as an official member of Van Halen, and you can see that I am trying to look happy about it.

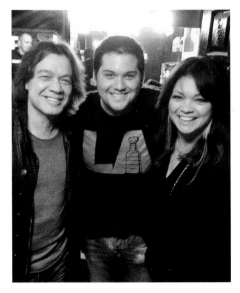

Wolfie was playing bass with Tremonti, and it was the first time Ed and I sat in the audience together and watched him play in front of a crowd. We kept squeezing each other all night.

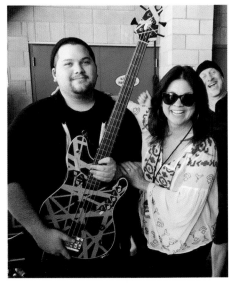

Before a Van Halen show. I am the proud mom, and Wolfie is wearing his "I'm putting up with my mom" face.

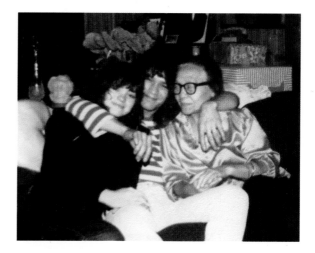

I know Mrs. Van Halen loved me, but look at the side-eye she's giving me.

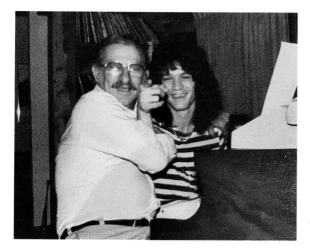

Mr. Van Halen and Ed at the piano that I still have.

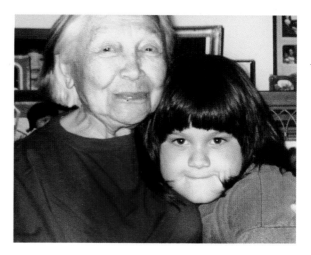

Wolfie and his "oma," Mrs. Van Halen.

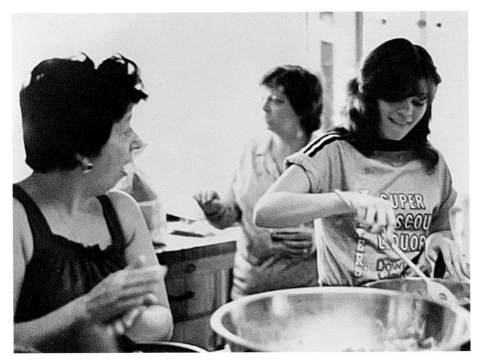

In the kitchen with Aunt Adeline and Aunt Norma the week before Ed and I got married. The whole family had come to LA, and we cooked and laughed together.

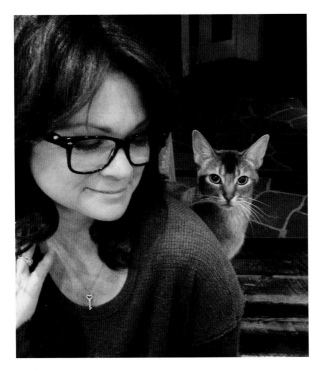

With my buddy Dexter, who is always watching over me.

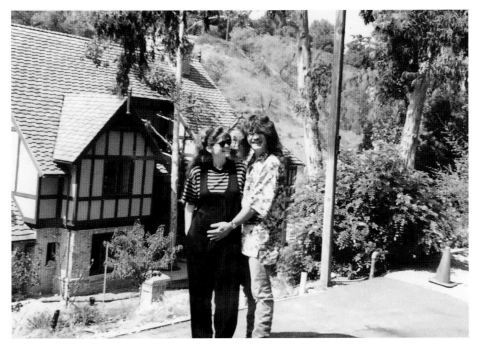

Pregnant and building our dream house. Ed was so happy; he couldn't wait for the baby to arrive.

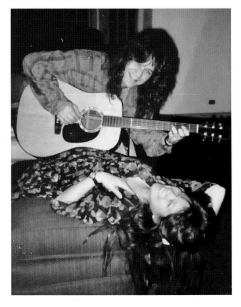

I am six months pregnant, and Ed is playing the song that would become "316" on my belly.

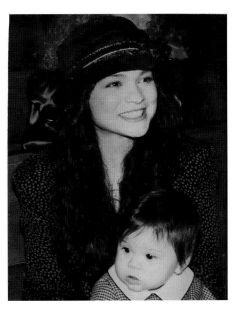

Me and Wolfie. He's a little less than a year old.

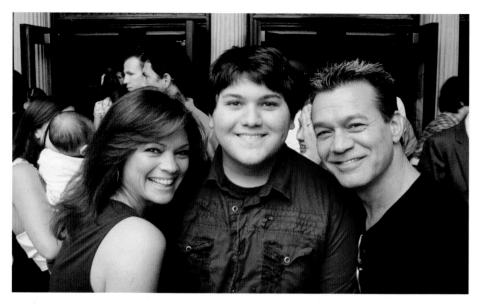

The proud parents at Wolfie's high school graduation.

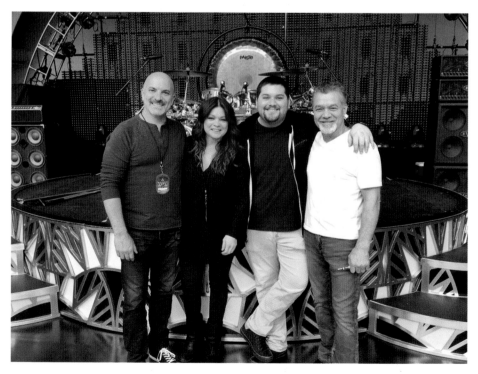

At the Hollywood Bowl before the Van Halen show in 2015. We didn't know it then, but this turned out to be one of the last two shows the band played. My dream was always to see Ed play the Hollywood Bowl, and he did it with Wolfie.

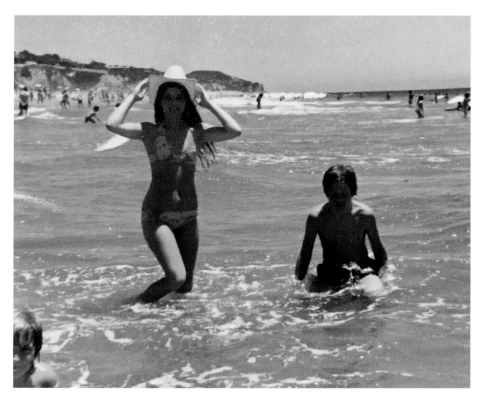

At Zuma Beach in 1975 with my brothers, Patrick and David, and I wish I could tell that fifteen-year-old girl she's perfect the way she is.

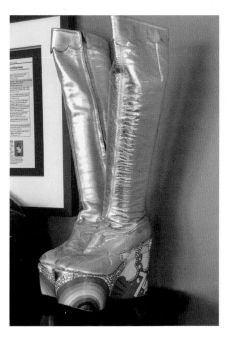

The famous Elton John boots I wore on *One Day at a Time*.

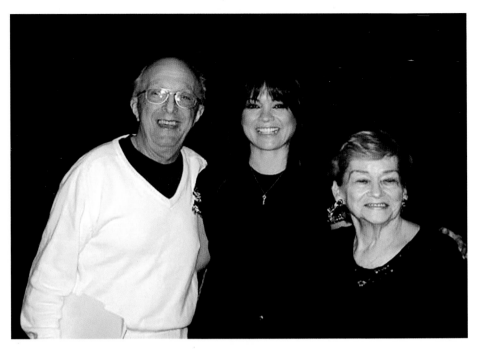

The theater in Wilmington with my parents, who came to see me give a talk, after which we all went to my Aunt Adeline's for dinner.

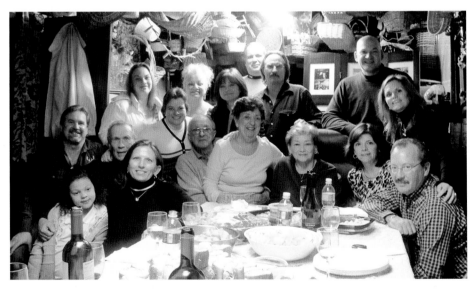

The extended Bertinelli family in my Aunt Adeline's basement kitchen, which inspired all of my cooking dreams.

# A Room with a View

LATE SPRING–SUMMER 2020

I HAVE NEVER BEEN ONE of those people who decorates my house like a museum or a movie set, where each item is curated to look camera-ready in case *Architectural Digest* knocks on the door unannounced for a photo shoot. My house is distinctly and intentionally comfortable. Blame it on my upbringing. Some people are formal. I am not. I grew up wearing flip-flops and faded blue jeans and T-shirts (the one I have on now is bleached maroon and says PEACE across the front), and my house has that same casual style.

My cats and dog have free run of the place. I have a grown-up kid who still shows up with friends, counting on me to have a well-stocked fridge. Most days I am working at the kitchen table, which is cluttered with stacks of cookbooks, magazines, newspaper clippings, notes, mail, reminders, to-do lists, and other evidence that I move slower than the rest of the world.

I prefer going at my own pace. Back in my twenties, I tried the fast lane. Since then, I have discovered that I am much better managing from the right side of the road. Actually, I am best when the car is parked in the garage and I can be right here at home, which, I have come to realize, is a project that parallels the work I have done (or not done) and continue to do on myself. It hasn't been without its complications and procrastinations, indecisions and expenses, but I have gotten myself to a place that I really, really like.

Some people do this with a house or a garden or a car—something that reflects who they are at that point in time and the work they are constantly doing on themselves. Ed is like that; in addition to his talent as a musician, he has the mind of an engineer. He has frequently called himself a tinkerer, a handy do-it-yourself trait he inherited from his dad, who was also a musician. Mr. Van Halen played the clarinet and saxophone, and once had to adapt the latter instrument after he lost part of a finger while trying to move a neighbor's U-Haul trailer off its jacks and out of his way at three in the morning.

Don't ask. It's typical Van Halen family lore—equal parts macho, alcohol, and ingenuity. Well, maybe not equal parts.

Ed started building and tearing apart guitars when he was in high school. He holds two United States patents, numbers 4656917 and 388117. The first was for a smoother neck that helped him play his trademark tapping style and the other was for an improved guitar peghead that made restringing easier. In 2015, he wrote about both in *Popular Mechanics.* He had a workshop in his studio that was like something you'd see on *This Old House;* it was so cluttered with dozens of projects in various states that he could've had his own show called *This Old Guitar.* He saved every piece of equipment and could tell you how many drops of 3-IN-ONE oil he put in the nut of a whammy bar he rebuilt in the seventies.

I remember an MTV News interview he did with Chris Connelly in the late nineties where he gave a tour of the studio. We hadn't split yet, and I remember the 5150 studio well. It looked similar to one of those places you see on *American Pickers* where stuff is piled floor to ceiling and only the owner knows the where-abouts of things. To get around the city code, he had built a rac-quetball court and turned it into his personal playhouse. As he gave Chris the tour, they came upon shelves of tapes, what looked like hundreds of them, at least hundreds of hours of music, a life-time of music, really.

Chuckling, Ed explained that all the tapes had been numbered and the contents catalogued on a Radio Shack computer that had broken down. Efforts to recover the info all proved unsuccessful. Ed said that he was the only one who could index what was on them. He recalled pulling down a tape from 1983 that had the song "Right Now" on it; that classic was released eight years later in 1991. He shrugged and said that he would go through them some day.

I don't know if that day ever came. But his relentless pursuit of perfection—whether making music, working on his instruments, or remembering what he had created and figuring out how and when to use it—has driven and defined Ed for as long as I have known him, and it was that way before I met him, too.

My mom was similar but in a different way. She was a wonder-ful artist, a painter who lost herself in her canvases. After all of us kids were grown, she worked as a travel agent, which was like painting landscapes. She enjoyed helping people plan their trips. She listened to their reasons for travel: some trips were for busi-ness, some were family vacations, some were much-needed get-aways amid crises. I think her work, like her art, was a kind of therapeutic escape that unlocked her imagination and allowed her access to a place where she eventually came to terms with the trag-edy of losing her second-born child.

My house has been my way of getting inside myself. For nearly twenty years, it has reflected who I am at the time and provided me with an opportunity to reimagine, fix, and change. It has become a place where I can relax and enjoy my surroundings. It has reminded me that I am strong. It has let me see myself as a work in progress. It has reminded me when something needs to be repaired and when I should stand still and admire beauty. It has given me roots and the courage to tear down and rebuild. It has gifted me with perspective.

· · · · · · · · ·

It doesn't have to be a house. It can be a single room. It can also be a car, a park bench, a public garden, a guitar, a painting. For me, it was my house. We literally grew into each other.

I began looking at homes after deciding that I was going to leave Ed. Dividing our property and assets was amicable and relatively easy. Finding a new home wasn't. Every day I drove around nearby neighborhoods looking at FOR SALE signs. I had some basic parameters, starting with affordability and location. I had a budget. I wanted to be near Ed for Wolfie's sake. I wanted to stay close to Wolfie's school. And I wanted privacy.

Then I looked for those intangibles, the mysterious qualities in a home that invited me in and promised comfort. The house I had left was a dream house. I had worked with architects to create everything Ed and I thought we wanted: enough bedrooms for three to four kids, tons of closet space, and ample room for our busy lives. We ended up with so much room that we led separate lives. Now I simply wanted a home that would allow me to settle in, gather my thoughts, figure out what was next, and help raise my child.

I found the house that became mine while driving through the hills slightly east of Ed's house. I had gone past Coldwater and Laurel Canyons, turned off Mulholland Drive, and was meandering aimlessly along narrow winding streets when I spotted a tree up on a hill. I couldn't see the house. But the tree turned out to be a large, sturdy live oak with sweeping branches that, upon a closer look, seemed like they were accessible and offering a lift up, which was what I needed. I also thought Wolfie would have so much fun climbing the tree. I think he probably climbed it twice.

Still, I bought the tree and stayed for the house. Like me, the house was not in great shape. There was water damage. Decks were broken. Stairs were loose. There were three porches—one off the kitchen, one off the living room, and one off the TV room—and all three were in various stages of falling apart. The house had four bedrooms, two on each side, and I liked that Wolfie and I could nestle in rooms on one end and I could use those on the other end as an office and a guest room. If any single feature made me feel like this was going to be my new home, though, it was the kitchen. It sat smack in the center of the house, which made sense to me. What was more central to daily life than a kitchen?

Though it had not been updated into one of those sparkling industrial workplaces with a farmhouse patina that was so pop- ular at the time, it was spacious and warm and immediately re- minded me of the kind of kitchen my Nonnie and Aunt Adeline would approve of. The appliances were laid out efficiently around a large center island; I could picture the two of them rolling out pasta dough there as they had done in my Aunt Adeline's basement in Delaware. Later on, I would cook there with my mom. I don't know if the best decisions are made in the gut, but the tastiest most certainly are.

One thing I was clear about: the large picture window at the far end of the kitchen. The house was perched on the side of a hill and the view out that window stretched forever. I could look across the entire valley and see the homes and stores below, the traffic on the freeway, the Burbank skyline, the planes on their way to Bob Hope Airport, and the mountains in the distance. Light poured through the glass, and at night the stars floated as if they were snacks in a celestial pantry. I needed that light and those stars, the view and all the space in between.

· · · · · · · · ·

The first person I showed it to was Ed. I wanted him to see that it was safe for Wolfie and me. He loved it and gave me a thumbs-up.

We moved in and lived in the house for about five years before I started to give serious thought to making some improvements. It kind of paralleled my life, the way I gained weight and stewed about it for years, and gained even more weight until finally I signed up for Jenny Craig. I was the same way with the house. I saw the deck falling apart, made a note about taking care of it, and three years later it was so eaten away by dry rot and bugs that I couldn't stand on it without risking injury.

One day, as I walked around the backyard, I decided I'd had enough of this obstacle course. I decided to take action. *If I'm going to fix the one deck*, I said to myself, *I might as well fix all of them*. It turned out to be the season for fixing things. Ed and I divorced so he could get remarried. Tom and I got engaged and planned our own wedding. Wolfie went on the road with Van Halen. With so much in flux, why not remodel the whole house, too?

That's the way I roll. Delay until the little things add up to the whole thing. But change also creates its own momentum, and I was swept up in the potential and excitement. I talked with my architect about building an upstairs master bedroom — my eagle's nest — to take advantage of the view and revamping the swimming pool. I was good with the living and dining rooms as they were, but I saw an opportunity to enlarge the kitchen and update the cabinets and appliances to make it the type of cooking area that I'd always envisioned.

Everything felt right, like a necessary next step. The decks were about giving myself safe, secure footing. The second-story bedroom was about letting my spirit soar. The kitchen was about feeding my soul. And the swimming pool, which I found myself enjoying in my dreams, was about giving myself a fresh start and new beginnings.

One piece of the puzzle left me, well, puzzled. That was my bedroom closet. I thought I wanted a large new closet, one of those closets I saw in magazines that looked like a secret apartment. You opened the door and saw an oasis of opulence and organization. But was that me? I am not a shopper. I am a T-shirt and jeans person. Maybe I should do a major cleaning out of what I have and go the opposite way, a more modest closet. I could do a meditation nook. An upstairs coffee bar. A reading corner.

Then I saw my Wallabees and put a stop to any and all fifty sides of my fantasies. Who was I kidding? I was a pack rat. I also saw the knee-high silver platform boots that I wore on the *One Day at a Time* episode where Mackenzie and I dressed up as Elton John and Kiki Dee, and sang their hit "Don't Go Breaking My Heart." Though I hadn't worn those boots since we shot that episode in 1976, I shut the closet doors and emailed my architect. "Forget what I said earlier. The closet has to be large."

After that *One Day* episode aired, Elton sent me an autographed picture that said I was a better Elton John than he was. I have had it reframed twice. It's one of my treasures. So there is a chance that I am just a big old softie rather than a hoarder. One thing about me was unchanged, though. I still moved at my own pace. The blueprints for all this lived on my dining-room table for about three years.

Finally, we broke ground and I was extremely excited, though what I remember most about the early days of construction is that we moved out to the beach house I bought in the eighties, and for the next two years, I had an hour-and-a-half commute twice a day from there to the studio where we shot *Hot in Cleveland* all the while knowing my real house was exactly one mile — or about ten minutes — from the set.

I suppose it added to the anticipation.

. . . . . . . . .

As work continued, I had two additions. I wanted a garden — a productive and edible garden. I missed the one I'd had up at Ed's house. I was very particular. I pictured fruit trees and became consumed about having a variety of them: orange, lemon, lime, grapefruit, guava, kumquat, avocado, and any other trees my genius gardener, Carlos, thought would grow. I also envisioned vegetables, hedges of rosemary, and clusters of other herbs.

All of a sudden, I was like my mom and Ed, tinkering with the yard. I was finally emerging from the depression over my first marriage ending and the ensuing uncertainty of who I was supposed to be at this stage of my life, and the garden reflected this. It was important to me. I was ready to be productive, fruitful, nourishing, and fresh — all the things I saw in a garden. I was also ready to have a new relationship with food. Rather than avoid it, I wanted to grow it. I wanted to be involved in the process. I had gone to Italy. I had written a cookbook. I had fallen in love with enjoying everything about a meal.

I didn't just eat the ingredients, I also savored them. I didn't need to know the provenance of my carrots and peas, but I wanted to appreciate the freshness and care that went into preparing the food. I saw myself harvesting the bounty in my yard, bringing it inside my kitchen, and preparing simple but delicious dishes for family and friends.

Dieting didn't cross my mind; engaging in something creative and warm and personal did. This was not about restriction or denial; it was about leaning forward and embracing something I had previously considered bad or off-limits. I wasn't even conscious of this change. I was acting on instinct. My body was telling me to eat; my soul was telling me to grow.

The garden took several years to plant and longer before it began producing fruit and vegetables in abundance. That was a good thing. I needed to learn patience and get into the routine of giving the garden daily attention and care, something I needed to work on with myself, too. And that was and still is the most valuable takeaway.

Happiness and joy are the fruits of a healthy life, but it takes work every day. My garden reminds me of this. You have to get your hands dirty.

The other feature I monitored during construction was a library. In some ways, this room might have triggered the whole remodel, more so than the broken decks. The library is actually a nook with floor-to-almost-ceiling bookshelves and a comfortable chair where I can plant my butt and read and stare out at the beautiful view. It's a cozy, comfortable hideout where I am able to *see* the quiet, stillness, and wonder of just being.

I have friends who meditate. They encouraged me to buy a meditation chair. I did and put it in my bedroom, where it is a landing spot for sweaters and T-shirts.

I meditate when I look up from a book or a crossword puzzle and gaze out the window for five or ten or even twenty minutes at a stretch. As I sort through a thousand different thoughts, I eventually find myself thinking of how beautiful everything is until I realize that I have cleared my mind and am thinking of nothing. I have watched birds soar and the sky fill with smoke from unchecked fires. I have floated across the sky on fluffy clouds and spied on deer feeding on my beloved garden.

I have sat here and thought about my parents as they aged and eventually succumbed to illnesses. I have been able to feel their presence even after they were gone. I have thought about my brother who died. Even though I never knew him, I have pictured him as a toddler. I have thought about my own son as he has grown up, graduated, and moved out on his own. I have laughed, cried, and worried. I have thought about my own good fortune and all the blessings that surround me and wondered why I still have such a hard time feeling good about myself. I have thought about Ed and his cancer. I have looked out at the sky during the day and at night, and prayed for him to beat it. I have asked God why.

Lately, I have caught myself thinking about what might be next, what that will be like for Ed, for Wolfie, and for all of us. What will that be like? What will that feel like?

I have looked for answers in the clouds and the stars. I have searched the mountains and the trees. I have watched them change and felt the timelessness of the big picture. I have sensed the way we pass through, mere visitors, and the way seeing ourselves in that manner prioritizes and reprioritizes things.

I sit here and marvel at the world's beauty and its flaws, and I think that I need to start looking at myself that same way: with respect and awe for all the pieces in the remarkable puzzle that is me and my life, including those pieces that don't seem to fit.

I have come to the conclusion that a room with a view is essential to happiness. But you don't need one like mine. Everybody has their own. It's called the human heart. There is no better window through which to look at yourself and the world than a full, warm, forgiving, aching, healing, and loving heart.

The other day I caught myself thinking about a secret little area in the garden near the oak tree where I put a bench. I haven't sat on it for months, but I like knowing it's there, waiting for me to arrive, as I have been doing most of my life—waiting for me to arrive.

I am getting there.

Definitely.

I'm getting there.

# The Twenty-One Gram Diet

## MARCH 2020

HAVE JUST FINISHED A question-and-answer session with a class of fourth graders. My cohosting duties on the Food Network's *Kids Baking Championship* has made me popular with this age group, and I gave these kids permission to ask me anything. However, the first question — *What four adjectives best describe you?* — made me wish I hadn't been so casual about the defining parameters.

Don't laugh. The problem was that I momentarily couldn't remember the difference between an adjective and an adverb.

That was lightweight stuff compared to when a girl asked what made me happy. Leave it to a kid to cut right to the chase.

I couldn't say, "Well, shoot, I've been asking myself that same question for years, especially lately." But I came close. I considered explaining that these things seemed to have changed depending on my age, whether I was nine years old like them, or in my twenties or thirties, or at my present age of sixty. However, as various answers came to mind, I realized that the things that make me happy, truly happy, haven't changed at all over the years: a hug from my son, a grilled cheese sandwich on a rainy day, reading a good book, seeing one of my cats napping on the windowsill, pretty flowers, falling asleep outside while I am reading, the fresh air in spring and fall, a walk along the beach, laughing till I have to run to the bathroom . . .

If anything, I explained to the kids, the list hasn't changed as much as it has expanded to include seeing my son in love, getting a surprise text from Ed, feeling healthy, learning a new tip or trick from one of my insanely talented chef friends . . . stuff like that.

Later, it crosses my mind that I didn't say that being thin or weighing less makes me happy. It never entered my mind. How about that, huh? *Food for thought,* I think.

Years of dieting and cleansing and the like has left me hungry, and what I'm hungry for can't be found in the refrigerator or pantry. What I want is for my soul to be fed with compassion, forgiveness, gratitude, kindness, and love. This is what I am talking about when I say that the joy I want to feel is not so much an end goal as it is a value and an intention that I have to realign with over and over again.

Joy is not going to come to me. I have to intentionally pursue it every day. I know I am repeating myself. But that's what it takes. Constant reminding. Joy, happiness, and gratitude have to be pursued. They don't automatically find us. We have to find them. I feel the same way about feeding my soul. I have to be intentional about it. Every day. The way I try to sit in the sun with a book for a few minutes or stare out at the vista from my kitchen window and marvel at the beauty of the mountains in the distance or literally stop to smell the roses. This is food for the soul. It's necessary for my well-being. It's something all of us need and crave, I think.

Where is this diet? Where is an easy-to-follow recipe for feeding our souls so our stomachs don't constantly tell us that we're hungry? How do we eat to feel good rather than eat so we don't feel?

I have come up with a seven-day program to nourish the soul. It's my Twenty-One Gram Diet.

At the moment we die, we supposedly weigh twenty-one grams less than we did when our heart was still pumping blood to our extremities and our bodies were still drawing breaths. The twenty-one grams is said to be the weight of our soul. This has helped me to arrive at a powerful realization: No matter how much weight I lose, I still feel heavy. But when my soul is nourished, I feel lighter no matter what the number is on the scale.

So have I and everybody else who has started a diet or a cleanse been going about this the wrong way? Have we been brainwashed into ignoring logic? Shouldn't we be feeding our souls rather than trying to shrink our waistlines?

Consider this: Things that weigh ten pounds include a small dog, a mini microwave, a bowling ball, a large bag of sugar, a sack of potatoes, and three two-liter bottles of soda. Things that weigh one gram include a paper clip, a quarter teaspoon of sugar, a thumbtack, a piece of gum, any US bill. It should be easier to add a paper clip than lose a mini microwave.

This is not a replacement for morning affirmations, ten-minute sun salutations, breathing exercises, stretching, yoga, meditation, absorbing the energy from crystals, or spoiling yourself silly by starting your day with a delicious omelet if that's what you are into. If you want to skip dessert or yell at or with Rachel Maddow, go ahead. I am not trying to interfere.

What I am suggesting is that you adopt this diet as an addition to your daily routine. Like you do when you take your vitamins, carve out at least a few minutes every day for this diet. You can spend more time on it if you have it, but keep in mind that the goal is to make sure your soul is full.

## Day One: Permission

On the first day of the Twenty-One Gram Diet, give yourself permission to feel good and see all your good, wonderful, and positive qualities instead of focusing on the things you consider shortcomings, flaws, and imperfections. Give yourself permission to turn off the news and turn on something you enjoy. Give yourself permission to play your favorite music, take a walk, call a friend, read a good book or even a trashy magazine. Give yourself permission to step out of your comfort zone and do something crazy. Or give yourself permission to cozy up inside your comfort zone and chill. Give yourself permission to expand rather than contract.

## Day Two: Compassion

On the second day, recognize the struggle and suffering you have endured for years. The battle to feel good about yourself and see yourself as unique and attractive and deserving of love and affection when you have spent years and maybe most of your life telling yourself that you are not worthy or a failure or labeling yourself as bad or fat or ugly or unlovable is real. The pain is real. Acknowledge it. Cry if you need to. Go back to the original source of the hurt. You may never have told anyone about it, but you know what it is. Or maybe you don't know what it is, but the feeling is there. Replay it in your mind. See yourself. See the incident for what it was. Recognize that you have spent a lifetime judging yourself because of it. This judgment has influenced your behavior. It hasn't just been unhealthy. It has also been unkind, unnecessary, and unproductive. Now say, "Enough already." Going forward, treat yourself with compassion and understand that you aren't perfect—and that nobody else is perfect, either. That's what it means to be human. Everyone carries around some form of hurt and suffering. Take time to treat everyone the way you want to be treated: with compassion. And treat yourself that way, too.

## Day Three: Forgiveness

I remember hearing Maya Angelou refer to forgiveness as a gift. "Forgive everybody," she said. I know what she meant when she called it "one of the greatest gifts you can give yourself." To me, forgiveness is the way we shine light on the darkness. On day three, give yourself this gift. Forgive yourself. Allow yourself the grace of space. When you forgive, you free yourself from the anger, hurt, blame, foolishness, criticism, and stupidity that you carry around inside. By letting go, you actually feel lighter. I work at this, and I have experienced the lightness that comes from forgiving people, and especially from forgiving myself, so I keep working at it. Little by little, I chip away at that big wall of blame and hurt that has encircled me. It opens me up. It lets in the light. It gets rid of the darkness.

## Day Four: Gratitude

On the fourth day, take time to stop and think about everything you have as opposed to everything you don't have, starting with the miracle that we exist and the opportunity that this provides us to experience what I think is the best part of being human—giving and receiving love and affection. My role model is Betty White. I have never seen or met anyone more full of gratitude than my former *Hot in Cleveland* costar. She greets each day with an appreciation of everything she has been through and an enthusiasm for the day, including her two favorite indulgences, vodka and hot dogs. The woman literally glows. Take your cues from her. Be grateful for your health. Be grateful for having enough to eat and maybe, I hope, having some to share. Be grateful for having a home to keep you warm and safe. Be grateful for the chance to help someone else experience the same things. Think about the last time you laughed and loved. You're smiling now. Everything else is gravy.

## Day Five: Kindness

Remember the way you smiled the day before? On the fifth day, do something that puts that same kind of smile on someone else.

## Day Six: Joy

On the sixth day, step outside—literally outside—and outside of yourself. Experience other people, the world, the universe. You will have to figure out the specifics for yourself, but that is what I try to do. I try to turn off everything in my head that says, *Me, me, me;* and if I truly make the effort and am lucky and alert, I will inevitably feel joy.

## Day Seven: Love

If you make the effort on the previous six days, the seventh will be effortless. You will have added the weight of a paper clip and feel like you lost a mini microwave. Without having to do anything, love will find you. *Love enters an open heart, and when you do this for six days, love will enter. And there's a danger in this. Once in a while, you will feel hurt. But as I am learning, the love is there more often than not.*

## Disclaimer

I make no promises. I offer no before and after pictures as evidence that this diet will put you in a smaller dress size. But it will put you in a better frame of mind. It does me. While I am far from perfect and my days can suck just like anybody else's, and I still hate sitting in front of my magnifying mirror when I pluck my eyebrows, I am learning that by intentionally practicing these values, one per day, I am usually able to treat myself better and love others more and open myself up to the possibility of experiencing joy immediately. In this moment. At this age. In this body.

*That's* what I want to feel.

# Bubba and Beau

## SPRING 2020

AM MORE UPSET ABOUT the possibility of losing Ed than I was after my parents died. I know that sounds terrible. I loved my parents. But my connection to Ed is different. The idea of never again being able to share a thought that only he would understand or ask him a question that only he would know the answer to or trade smiles across a room as we watch our son appear onstage in front of an audience that wants to see him just . . . well . . . that kind of loss scares me in a way that is indescribable.

When Van Halen was on tour in 2015, I believed Ed was going to beat cancer and be okay. He had battled the disease in various parts of his tongue and throat for a decade and a half. He had the best medical care available. Early on, of course, he could have helped himself by stopping smoking and drinking. You don't spit at cancer. You don't taunt the Big C. You don't pretend you can outrun it.

But Ed eventually moved past denial and anger and got his shit together. He took care of himself, and it showed. He looked and felt good. Then he had the motorcycle accident and learned that the cancer had spread throughout his body like a greedy developer run amok. Still, we remained hopeful, trusted the treatments, and clung to promising checkups. Sober in every way, he was upbeat, loving, and appreciative.

He is that way even now. Hopeful.

We texted the other day. Like everyone else, he was looking for a new TV series, and he wanted to know if I had any recommendations. Netflix, Amazon Prime, HBO—that's all anyone seems to talk about these days.

This pandemic is making all of us shut-ins.

I never thought of my parents as getting old or sick until suddenly they were. Though my mother was slowed in her forties by rheumatoid arthritis, which got progressively worse over the years, both of my parents easily cruised past age sixty-five. After my dad retired—he spent thirty-two years at General Motors—they moved to Las Vegas. "No state income tax," he explained. My dad was a Fox News devotee who made me more of a feminist than my mother or any book, TV show, movie, documentary, or person I heard speak could have done. I think he knew that and took pride in having a strong, independent daughter who could provide for herself.

But we generally avoided talking about politics and deeply personal stuff, preferring to keep conversations light and on the surface. There were too many booby traps. My dad was a responsible provider and loving father, but he was not a faithful husband, something that left scars on all of us. Football was a much safer topic when we gathered around the table. Growing up, all my brothers played, my dad assisted the coaches, and my mom and I turned into Sunday and Monday night die-hards who were as familiar with sweeps, draws, and sacks as we were with the latest Bloomingdale's catalog. That never changed.

In 2004, my parents moved to Scottsdale, Arizona. My youngest brother, Patrick, who lived in Scottsdale with his wife, Stacy, saw that they were slowing down. Because he and Stacy were the ones checking on them most frequently, he said that it would be easier if my parents were closer to them. We helped my parents find a beautiful house and they spent about ten years enjoying the dry desert air before a series of small heart attacks and related health issues took the steam out of my dad.

Then one day he took my mom to a doctor's appointment and the nurse at the front desk, who knew my parents well, became alarmed as soon as she saw him. He said that he felt tired. She hurried him into an examining room where it turned out that he was having a heart attack at that very moment. The nurse saved his life.

As he recovered, we were sad, scared, and realistic. This was the next unavoidable stage of adulthood, the one where you become the guardian of your own parents. My brothers and I talked and asked one another the questions that so many of our friends and people our age seemed to also be asking themselves: Can Mom and Dad take care of themselves? What do we do? How can we help?

· · · · · · · · · ·

It's one of those things you never really think about. It's not like when you are growing up and you spend a lot of time thinking about what it will be like to get your driver's license, live in your own apartment, have sex, get married, and have a baby. Then your parents get sick or stumble or begin to forget, and suddenly their care is all you think about.

Patrick and Stacy took the lead and I provided whatever additional support was needed. My parents were fortunate to have the resources to provide themselves with good options. We found a cheerful one-bedroom apartment in a comfortable assisted-living facility. Going through their belongings, accumulated over sixty-one years of marriage, was predictably emotional since we had to decide what to keep, what to donate, and what to toss; and almost every item had some kind of story or personal attachment to it.

Furniture was easy. It either fit into their new apartment or it didn't. If it didn't fit, the four of us talked through who wanted it or what to do if there were no takers. Appliances, electronics, pictures, and so on were handled similarly. The task spurred thoughts not just of what gets collected over a lifetime and what is necessary to make a life and raise a family, but also how we children broke away from our parents and created our own lives. Was I really only eighteen when I bought my first house? And just on the cusp of twenty-one when I got married?

My dad was super organized and had everything in boxes that were clearly labeled. We found deeds and contracts for our old homes. School art projects and reports were in folders. There was an old baby book for my brother, Mark, including congratulatory cards from relatives and friends stuck in the front of the book, which, of course, ended abruptly and was, I assumed, put away until we found it again.

That wasn't the only sensitive family subject we unearthed. While sifting through boxes and albums of photos and documents, we unearthed a handwritten letter from my dad's half brother whom we had never heard about. We knew Nazzareno had traveled to America, met my grandmother, and had three children — my dad and his two sisters, Norma and Adeline — but we had no idea that he had deserted a whole other family in Italy. It was a genuine "holy shit" discovery.

"Dear Andrew," the letter began. "It's your brother Ernesto that is writing to you. I think you know our history. Our father went to America when I was 3 and left me in Italy. He wrote me and I know that you are my true brother. I have a great wish, that is to see you personally."

We wondered whether they had ever met and ultimately concluded that they hadn't. But who knew? We decided not to bring it up with Dad. What was the point other than to know—and now we knew. But I saw a similarity between Nazzareno and my dad. Both had secrets, including some that had impacted their families. The two of them were like old-fashioned Italian restaurants: white tablecloths; stiff cloth napkins; the smell of garlic wafting from the kitchen; a menu with classic antipasto, fried calamari, spaghetti marinara, fettucine alfredo; and a back room where stuff happened that nobody knew about.

I wasn't suddenly ready to forgive my dad, but I understood him better. When it came to being a husband, he didn't have the most virtuous teacher.

·········

One of our prerequisites for the move was making sure that their cat, Beau, could go with them to the assisted-living center. They were very attached to him. At this point, my parents had only one of their two cats. Six months earlier, their other cat, Bubba, had gone missing. But as we were on our way to take one more look at the new apartment before signing the agreement, my cell phone rang. On the other end was a woman who asked if I had lost a cat.

"What do you mean?" I asked, thinking that Beau had escaped from the house because we had been going in and out so often.

"It's a white cat with an orange tail and blue eyes," the woman said. "But he looks like he's been out on the streets for a while."

Telling her to hold on for a second, I put the phone down and scratched my head. I had to think. Then it hit me.

"You didn't just find Bubba, did you?" I asked.

"Um, I don't know if it's Bubba," she said. "I found a cat that has clearly been abandoned."

"Where did you find him?" I asked.

She told me. When I mentioned that this was less than a mile away from my mom and dad's house, she got mad at me.

"This poor cat," she said. "We thought someone abandoned him . . . because, you know, a lot of people do. Unfortunately, they just don't want to take care of their cats anymore and they throw them into feral colonies."

"No, no, no, you don't understand," I said, explaining that we were heartbroken when we couldn't find Bubba and put up fliers everywhere.

It turned out that Bubba had been living behind the local grocery store, where the employees and the owner of the dry cleaner's next door kept him fed but couldn't grab him for six months. Once they got ahold of him, they had him scanned and called the number on file, which was my cell phone. Bubba was my dad's cat, and he was ecstatic to have him back. So was Beau. The four of them moved into the assisted-living facility. When I visited them a few days later, my parents were in bed and Bubba and Beau were curled up on the bed with them, like they'd never been apart.

My parents liked their routine at the assisted-living facility. One day my dad was downstairs being Mr. Helpful, as was his way, and he saw a woman who looked like she was about to fall. He hurried over to her side and caught her just as she lost her balance. He broke her fall, but she fell on top of him and broke his hip. He went downhill from there and never recovered.

I can't help but think of the old saying: It's not going to kill you to be nice. Except it did in his case. On December 7, 2016, only six weeks after that accident, he was gone. I have a picture of Bubba sitting on the bed with my dad after he drew his final breath. Dad was ready to go. His feline friend, though looking forlorn, was still offering comfort.

. . . . . . . . .

I mourned and grieved with the rest of my family until gradually the routine of talking to my parents and checking in on them became solely focused on my mom. Sadness came in waves. Concern for my mom filled the space between those waves. She was crushed after my dad passed. Whatever his shortcomings as a husband had been in the past, she had made her peace with them long ago and he had done the same, turning into a devoted caregiver as her rheumatoid arthritis limited her activities and filled her days with pain.

I am not sure why cruelty and compassion often walk hand in hand, and yet they do far too often. Are they two sides of the same coin? It doesn't make sense.

My mom had a tough life. A Jersey girl by birth, she was only nine years old when her mother died. Her stepmother was horrible, and I am pretty sure she was sexually abused as a teenager. She never explicitly said those words, but she dropped hints and made it clear she was eager to get out of her house. She met my dad one snowy winter night as she came out of a movie theater in Claymont, Delaware. As she waited for a bus, he pulled up in his car and offered her a ride home. She declined. He drove off but circled back and implored her to accept a ride rather than stand in the freezing weather.

Five months later, they were married. I wish that this had ended her hardships. Sadly, it didn't. During the first few years of their marriage, my dad's family treated her poorly because she wasn't Italian or Catholic. Then my brother Mark died, and my dad's family held that tragedy against her, too. Devastated, she coped by trying to be an even more attentive mother and wife. The gods were still not kind. My dad cheated on her. In her forties, she was diagnosed with rheumatoid arthritis and endured pain for the remainder of her life. She never got a break. What was the point?

I have always asked myself the same question about Mark. What was the point of his or any life if it is going to end that soon?

My poor mom. When I was eight or nine years old, she had a hysterectomy. One day she took me with her to a doctor's appointment. I suppose no one was able to watch me. I sat next to her in the front seat of the car. Every time she hit a bump in the road, she winced in pain, and then turned to me and apologized. For what? Why did she feel the need to say she was sorry when she was the one suffering? She did the same thing years later as her arthritis began crippling her. She did this even late in her life, as she began to fail. It made no sense.

I should have taken hold of her and apologized to her for all of the suffering she'd endured throughout her life and was continuing to deal with. I did tell her how wonderfully talented she was and how much I loved and appreciated her, and how I knew all the luck and largesse I enjoyed in my life would never have been possible if not for her giving birth to me, driving carpool, sitting on sets, putting her own desires and ambitions on hold to be a great mom.

But I wasn't able to have a deeply personal heart-to-heart with her. Not about losing my brother Mark. Not about my dad's cheating. Not about the arthritis. Not about the way the arthritis eventually forced her to quit painting. Not about the way it shrunk her life to weekly doctor's appointments and constant medication, and ultimately led to her being bedridden. I never said I understood or was sorry for everything she endured. I never said I get it, and if you need to cry, go ahead and cry.

Only once, back when I was in my late twenties, did she come close. We were arguing about something and she walked right up to the edge of revealing her pain, whatever it was at that moment, before I stopped her.

"Don't," I said. "Don't go there."

She looked at me in a way that I have never forgotten, and said, "Why don't you want to be close to me? Why can't we be close?"

It wasn't that I didn't want to be close or that we weren't close in other ways. It was that I didn't want to see her pain. I was scared of it, scared of what would happen if those wounds were opened. I didn't see how much both of us would have benefited from being more open and honest with each other. We wouldn't have had to carry around so much damn weight.

When I get bogged down by feelings and emotions, I isolate and shut down until I reach the point where I shrug and accept the negativity or pain as a part of me. "Well, that's just me." I was taught by the best.

This is the part I am attempting to change and let go of with the work I am doing now. I don't have to hide what's in my heart. I don't have to punish myself for things that happened ages ago. I don't have to suffer for behavior that was ingrained in me. And I don't have to always feel like there is something about me that I need to fix.

I am fine.

I am good.

I am bad.

I am broken.

I am perfect the way I am.

I am human.

I can do something my mother wasn't able to do. I can love myself. As I am. At this age. Right now.

It's enough already.

. . . . . . . . .

After my dad died, my mother lived three more years. Given how much pain she was often in, I sometimes wondered why she survived instead of him. Her back was gone, she'd had two knee operations, and she was always searching for the right recipe of drugs that would give her relief. It was almost like God kept her around to continue punishing her. She wasn't a Buddhist who believed life was about suffering. She was smart, beautiful, sensitive, funny, and very talented. Her situation left me completely bewildered. What was the point?

She seemed to relax after Dad was gone. When I visited her, I made sure Bubba and Beau were fed and clean and that their litter box was emptied, and we sat together and talked about the cats as if they were part of our family, which, of course, they were. We watched old movies. My mother loved the Katharine Hepburn movie *Summertime.* It took place in Venice, and we spoke about going back there even though she wasn't strong enough to travel to California, let alone fly across the ocean.

If I visited on a Sunday, we watched football together. She wore her red number 11 Arizona Cardinals jersey in honor of her favorite player, the great wide receiver Larry Fitzgerald, and I arrived in my number 9 Saints jersey with BREES printed on the back. One year she organized a Super Bowl party at the assisted-living facility.

I usually surprised her with a big bag of Cheetos, which she loved. I did, too. They brought back memories for me. When I was in high school, I took a little bag of Cheetos, a sandwich, and a can of Pepsi every day for lunch. So my mom and I reminisced —two chicks who had spent most of their lives dieting the way Thelma and Louise ran from the law were eating Cheetos and licking their fingers without guilt or shame.

What I realized with even more clarity was the way food was our bridge to talking and connecting in a way we never did before.

That's the way I found out my dad's family had been mean to her after my parents were first married and also how they eventually warmed up to her after she spent years standing alongside them in my Aunt Adeline's basement kitchen, listening to them talk about the family and the old country while making pasta. Basically, she was an English-Irish girl who had to convert to Italian.

Though she bore the scars of those painful experiences, at least she was able to laugh at them sixty years later. She won. She outlived all of them. And that's the ultimate prize. Waking up in the morning is the only way you get to see what happens next. It also gives you the last word if you want it. Only the living can write or rewrite history. But my mom didn't care two wits about revising anything, and I came to realize that the three years she survived without my dad enabled her to shed the burdens, slights, hurt, and criticisms of the past and simply exhale. Like me, she was able to say, "Enough already."

At least I hope so.

. . . . . . . . .

My mom passed away in her sleep on June 18, 2019, the day before what would have been her sixty-fifth wedding anniversary. She had fallen the year before and she had been mostly bedridden since January. Her body was slowly breaking and coming apart. Patrick and Stacy called to say that she was shutting down. I was confused, actually in denial of what I already knew was inevitable, and I asked how they knew. "You know," Patrick said.

When I got the call that she was gone, I was about to get up and go to work on season seven of *Kids Baking Championship*. I was relieved that she was finally out of pain and that her suffering was over. In the end, she had been in tremendous pain. I still went to work, because you don't not show up for work, and Ed reached me while I was in the makeup chair. Wolfie had told him about my mom, and we had a tearful talk.

Afterward, he texted me a picture of him with my mom. He has his arm around her. My mom is grinning at the camera and Ed is looking lovingly at her. He seemed more distraught than I was, and eventually I figured out why. Ed knew his cancer had spread, and he was processing the gravity of the diagnosis and the fight ahead of him. I still didn't know about his situation at that point —and either he wasn't ready to tell me or he had decided the timing wasn't right.

But my mom's passing hit both of us hard. It sent a message to both of us: Time does not wait for anyone. Don't waste it.

I am reminded of this every time I walk into my sunroom— or, as I call it, the "catio." There on the chair or in the cat tree are Bubba and Beau curled up together.

# Blessings

## JULY 2020

I T'S SUMMER — THE middle of July — and nothing is happening. Covid has shut everything down. Everyone is confused, scared, depressed, and anxious. Ordinarily, I would be traveling a couple of times a month to food festivals, speaking engagements, New York City, and maybe taking a vacation. But I have not gone anywhere or done much of anything.

I miss traveling. The more I am not in Italy, the more I want to be there. I also want to go to London. I just want to go. Somewhere.

In a few weeks, we are taping the new season of *Kids Baking Championship*. The Food Network has found a hotel an hour south of me in Palos Verdes where we can create our own bubble and shoot the episodes with everyone getting tested beforehand and wearing masks throughout production. I am looking forward to getting back together with my pal, master baker Duff Goldman, the crew, and a new batch of talented kid bakers.

Actually, I am eager to be around other people again. I am hungry for conversation, laughter, stories, and cute pictures of children and pets. It has only been about a month or so since Wolfie and Andraia decided that it was safe to come inside the house when visiting me. The three of us were tired of waving and yelling through the windows. Our temperatures were normal, our hands were washed, rewashed, and wrinkled, and we were not going anyplace other than the grocery store. So I told them to come in. "The door is open."

"Hi, Ma!" Wolfie said.

My arms were already wide open and ready to grab him. We hugged. I didn't let go. It had been way too long. My eyes filled with tears. I could feel my soul inflate inside me. Never underestimate the power of a hug.

Since then, Wolfie has been coming over with more frequency, and those hugs are more important than ever. Between Covid and Ed, the backdrop has been so gloomy. The hugs reignite my sense of hope. My spirit lightens after each one. Forget those stickers on the back of cars that say MY CHILD IS AN HONOR STUDENT. I want one that says MY KID HUGS ME. It is a blessing—and like most blessings, it is delivered in a small package that is so ordinary looking it's easy to overlook or take it for granted.

You have to pay attention or else you are going to miss the joys in life. That has been my problem. I have not been paying attention.

It has been seven months since I went on the *Today* show and announced that I wanted to stop letting my concerns about my weight cast a negative shadow over everything in my life and to experience joy instead. As I was right then. In my body. At my age. I didn't want to always think I had to fix something about myself. It was enough already. As I told Angie Johnsey, the mind coach the *Today* show introduced to me, I sensed that I would find I wasn't all that broken if only I could get myself to see more of the good.

Either that or everybody is kind of broken, and being kind of broken is actually normal and okay.

Angie worked with me on recognizing the voices in my head that spoke to me, especially the one that always said I needed to lose ten pounds before I could even begin to think of myself as being on the right track. Then Covid hit. The world went full stop.

I turned sixty.

Ed's battle with cancer took a turn none of us had wanted to imagine.

I didn't see my son in person for months.

I didn't see anyone for months.

Life got very slow. Clothes were closeted in lieu of sweats and pj's. Every day was Tuesday or Wednesday or Friday or Saturday. It didn't matter. But the cats purred and stretched out in the sunlight. The dog chased the squirrels. The flowers bloomed. Fruit appeared on the trees. The orange blossoms and jasmine perfumed the air. I enjoyed the warmth of the sun. I basked in the quiet. And in the very stillness that surrounded me, I did the thing that had somehow eluded me for so long. I began to count my blessings.

I didn't even have to work at it. One day I thought of the delicious simplicity of a bologna sandwich, like the kind I took for lunch in elementary school. Two slices of Oscar Mayer bologna, Wonder Bread, and mayonnaise. I loved them — the taste; the soft white bread; the gooey, buttery sweetness of the mayo; and the tenderness of the bologna slices.

You know what? As I remembered those sandwiches, I found myself grinning from ear to ear.

It was a blessing — a blessing that I had parents, a family, and a mom who packed my lunch, and that I wasn't hungry.

Later, I thought of my sweet cat Dexter, who had passed away years ago at thirteen from cancer. He was nestled by my side through the hardest years of my life. A blessing.

A few days went by, and out of the blue I was picturing myself in a helicopter seated next to Ed and flying into Devore, California, for the US Festival. It was May 1983, and Van Halen was headlining the heavy metal portion of the three-day concert in the desert that was the brainchild of Apple cofounder Steve Wozniak. As the pilot zeroed in on his landing spot, we swept over the massive sea of people below us, several hundred thousand metal fans partying to Mötley Crüe, Ozzy Osbourne, and other bands, while eagerly anticipating Ed and company. I remember Ed shaking his head in awe and chuckling from nerves and disbelief. They played that night for two hours. Ed was adorable in overalls that matched the design of his Frankenstein guitar. David Lee Roth was obnoxiously brilliant. The whole experience was like a crazy dream, the craziest, wildest, best dream you could have.

Thirty-seven years later, I was in my backyard looking out at the wide-open view across the valley while picturing that scene, and all of a sudden laughter was seeping out of me. I shook my head the way Ed had in the helicopter. Disbelief. *Did that happen? Yes, that really happened. Oh my God.*

A blessing.

So here I sit today, right now, in sweats and a T-shirt, with no idea how much I weigh and no intention of getting on a scale this week or next.

Yes, I could lose ten pounds, and I wouldn't complain if I lost twenty, but my outlook is not dependent on it. I don't need to fit into a bikini. Physically, my goal as of this moment is to be healthy enough when I am eighty to climb the stairs to my bedroom without assistance or breathing heavily. Obviously, I am more of a realist than an overachiever. In the meantime, I am still counting . . .

· · · · · · · · ·

Blessings:
My family.

Getting a job as young as I was on *One Day at a Time*, thanks to Norman Lear, the greatest producer in the history of television, whose track record could have made him an intimidating tyrant. But he turned out to be kind, gentle, nurturing, sweet, and loving.

Working with Bonnie Franklin, Pat Harrington, and Mackenzie Phillips. Each of them taught me lessons in their own way. Bonnie, so gifted, taught me the subtleties of acting. Mac, though only six months older than I was, had grown up much quicker and was a model of strength and wisdom and resiliency. And Pat taught me the art of timing.

Meeting Ed was a blessing.

Not having any social media at the time was also a blessing. Otherwise I probably would have posted some stupid things or been videoed behaving like an idiot and would still be paying for it today.

Wolfie.

*Hot in Cleveland* was a gift that turned into five years of pure joy. Do you hear that? I used the word "joy." Not just that. I called it *pure joy.*

And it was. The script came to me at the end of 2009. I had not heard of TV Land, the cable channel that was producing it, which had previously been a home to reruns and movies. But I was told that they were now producing their own original content. I read the script about three LA-based women working in show business whose plane to Paris makes an emergency landing in Cleveland, Ohio, where they decide to stay and rent a house that comes with an eccentric older caretaker living a full and active life despite her age.

I loved the script. I was told the show was talking to Jane Leeves and Wendie Malick and that Betty White had already been cast as the caretaker. Though I didn't know which part they wanted me to play, I heard the names of these other women, and said, "Okay, I'm in." I had no idea the producers were telling Jane and Wendie the same story and getting the same response. Everyone signed up. In February 2010, we had our first table read, which was magic, and we were on the air in June.

The five years I spent on that series were the best working years of my life. Jane had been one of my good friends since Faith Ford introduced us when Wolfie was a toddler. Wendie instantly became a close friend, too. And Betty White was exactly the way people imagine—funny and quick-witted, with an outlook that inspired me every day I was around her; the woman literally glowed. She was truly a light. And our guest stars—Carl Reiner, Mary Tyler Moore, Tim Conway, Cloris Leachman, Carol Burnett, Joan Rivers, and so many more—were a who's who of performers that turned me into a fangirl every week.

Blessings all—and too many more to count.

. . . . . . . . .

The month before my mother died, I won two Emmy Awards. Mom was not able to watch because the 2019 *Daytime Emmy Awards* were streamed live on Facebook instead of being shown on regular TV, and at her age and in her condition, that was more than she was able to handle. I called her with the good news afterward.

"I am so happy for you," she said. "You deserve it."

Did I? Was she right? In 1981, I won a Golden Globe for my work on *One Day at a Time.* In 1982, I won again for Best Supporting Actress in a Series. The first year I took my mom as my date. The next year Ed was with me. I remember being shocked both times. I don't remember anything else. An Internet search of those occasions only reminds me that life is a series of hairstyles that get less embarrassing as you get older, especially if you lived through the eighties. Somewhere in those blow-dried locks is a life lesson.

The Globes always sat on a bookshelf somewhere. After Ed and I redid our house, I put them in the library. Then they moved with me to my present house, where they rested on a shelf in my office at the back of the house. They made for nice bookends. Sometimes I saw them. Most of the time I paid no attention to them.

I always wanted an Emmy, though. It was something that meant your work was accepted and that your talent was respected by your peers, and deep down I was always searching for something that would provide the validation I wasn't able to feel on my own. When I watched the award shows, I would imagine what I would say if my name was ever called. I didn't want to be one of those people who read names off a list.

It turned out that I didn't have to worry. Despite numerous series and dozens of movies, I managed to squeeze by without a nomination. The pressure wasn't merely off. It was never on. I had fun, but I was able to tell myself that I wasn't any good. Then, after trading acting for an apron, I was nominated for not one but two Emmy awards.

I was truly shocked. I was about to shoot the ninth season of *Valerie's Home Cooking,* and even then, though I had shot nearly one hundred episodes, an equal number of short video tutorials, and grown more comfortable in the kitchen, I read and reread the online notification and the text messages that came in and kept asking myself, *Really?*

It was amazing, and no one was more amazed than I was. I still had so many days—way too many days—when I felt like an imposter. It wasn't that I was pretending or that I lacked the skills to do the job or that I wasn't working my ass off every day to always learn and improve. No, I was afraid some online troll would call me out for playing the part of a TV cook, and even though there was nothing disingenuous about my work in the kitchen, that one criticism, even if it was the lone negative comment out of a thousand compliments, always triggered a rash of self-doubt and upset me for days.

It was that old childhood gremlin, feeling that nothing was enough.

Feeling . . . not deserving.

I wish I had the willpower to ignore the comments in my social media. I know better and I still can't keep myself from looking at them. In general, they are overwhelmingly positive, friendly, and kind. They make me smile and feel as if I have amassed thousands of friends over the years. The sick part is that I search out the Negative Nellies as they are confirmation of the worst I think about myself. *Ah, they have seen the real me.*

Except the real me was in the tenth season of my cooking show, grateful for the nomination, and just maybe and quite probably deserving of it.

*Enjoy,* I told myself. On the day of the Emmys, I was 99 percent sure I wasn't going to win, so I was able to relax and enjoy getting dressed up and going to the party. My biggest worry was whether my pants were going to fit. Sound familiar to anyone? Earlier in the week, Lori, my stylist from the show, had brought over a black tuxedo jacket and pants for me to try on, had them altered, and brought them back. But things change. However, this was my lucky day. They fit.

I've known makeup artist Lisa Ashley and hair stylist Kimmie Urgel since our *Hot in Cleveland* days, and we've become friends, so hair and makeup were a breeze. That left one last concern: hoping that my shoes wouldn't be too painful and cause my feet to throb midway through the show. Did I worry about these things when I was twenty-three?

My husband Tom and I took a car to the theater with executive producers Jack Grossbart and Marc Schwartz, who was also my longtime manager. There I was, seated next to Giada, who was nominated in my same categories, and I thought, *I'm going to watch her go up and accept the award and I'm going to be okay with it because she deserves it. She's amazing.* Moments before the show began, I was moved to the aisle, where I sat next to *Jeopardy!* host Alex Trebek, who had once guested on *Hot in Cleveland* and was a very funny and kind man.

When it was time for my first category, Outstanding Culinary Program, Rachael Ray, a friend and early inspiration of mine, appeared onstage to read the nominees and announce the winner. I was thinking about how cool it would be if I won my very first Emmy and got it from Rachael, because I adored her and knew she would be very happy for me. I had even worked as a correspondent for her show. Then, in the brief pause before she read the winner's name, I saw the joy in her face and knew it was my turn, and I burst into tears.

I was in shock. Blinded by tears, I somehow made it up the stairs and onto the stage without tripping. Then, despite years of thinking about what I would say if I ever did get an Emmy, I realized that I did not have anything prepared. I was so sure I wasn't going to win that I didn't bother. What did come out of me was genuine disbelief, which I expressed succinctly in two words: "Holy [fill in the blank]." A few moments later, I picked up my second Emmy of the night for Best Culinary Host. I asked all of my producers to join me onstage, then I tried to thank everybody I could think of. No one does anything by themselves, and my big insight, in retrospect, is that gratitude is the staircase you climb to get to joy.

·········

The wins were followed by drinks that night and phone calls to my mom and brothers the next morning after my coffee and Advil kicked in. I did something unusual for me: I let myself bask in the validation bestowed by those statues, which I placed on the kitchen table, where they stood like superheroes ready to fend off an attack by the dreaded foe known as imposter syndrome. I let them buoy the faith I had in myself, as awards are wont to do, and gradually I stopped beating myself up and let belief and pride seep into my self-esteem. All the long hours, the learning, and my experience were paying off.

A few weeks later, I moved the Emmys onto the dining-room table so I could see them as soon as I walked through the front door. *Hello, Best Culinary Host. Welcome back, Best Culinary Program.*

. . . . . . . . .

Almost a year later, I moved the shiny statuary onto the top of a cabinet near the entry where they are not so in-your-face. I am able to see them, and they can see me, but other people don't need to wear sunglasses every time they come through the door.

A few more months go by, and just the other day, on a whim, I bring my two Golden Globes out from hiding and set them down next to the Emmys. Suddenly, there is a crowd on top of the cabinet, a gathering of cherished acquaintances old and new. *Emmys, meet my Golden Globes. Golden Globes, meet my Emmys.* I am proud of them and all they represent, and that is okay. Even better is the way I think about myself. I hear my mom's voice: "You deserve it."

Sometimes, maybe even most of the time now, I believe her. And that, let me tell you, is a blessing.

# My Mother's Recipe Box

## JULY 2020

EVEN THOUGH IT'S SUMMER and I should be making a light, warm-weather meal for dinner, I have a craving for lasagna. A recipe card titled MOM'S LASAGNA sits nearby on the counter, but I don't really need it. I pulled it out of the recipe box from habit. This is a dance I have done enough times to know the steps by heart. With deft movements, I get the onion and garlic going; add the ground beef, sweet Italian sausage, hot Italian sausage, and season them; then I move on to the *besciamella*, which is a twist I made to my mother's recipe ages ago much to her consternation.

The kitchen fills with the pungent garlicky aroma that I remember from our favorite restaurant in Florence, and my eyes involuntarily shut for a moment as I savor the flavor in the air. After a teaspoon of self-satisfied laughter, I quip to myself, *Hey, I should have my own cooking show.*

The lasagna noodles are next. But I am interrupted when the phone rings. It's a robocaller asking if I want to extend my car warranty. *Really? Now?* I don't know a single person who hasn't received this same call about forty times. None of us need our car warranties extended. *Attention robocallers—yes, you, all of you sell-ing warranties, telling me that my Social Security card has been stolen; warning me that someone has charged seven hundred dollars on my Amazon card, which I don't have; and so on—please stop.*

Enough already.

Still, the timing of the call is such that it could have easily been my mother calling from a world beyond ours to tell me that it's not really lasagna unless I use ricotta cheese. This is a disagreement we had for years and a point that she made to me regularly and with good-natured enjoyment as if we were debating two sides of a spending bill on CNN.

Except there was nothing to debate other than preference. There are only two issues with lasagna. One: Do you use ricotta or not? My mother said yes. I say no need. And two: Who gets the crispy corners? My mom and I agreed that this is the best part of any lasa-gna. It's often the source of family fights and secret picking before the dish gets to the table.

Am I right? I am always stunned when I hear about people who don't like this part. Are they also among those who push the cream-cheese frosting on carrot cake off to the side because they don't like it? That's a move I will never understand.

Can we agree that carrot cake, as delicious as it might be, is nothing more than a delivery system for cream-cheese frosting, which itself is a reminder of the sweet taste of your first kiss from your first crush?

Getting back on point, there is much more to lasagna than the four crispy corners. In a well-made lasagna, the flavors blend and mesh thoroughly during baking but still contain tiny pock-ets where the bite packs an intense burst of oregano or basil or a piece of wine-soaked sausage with a nugget of melted Parme-san attached like a salty barnacle. It's a dance down the Spanish Steps performed on your tongue, and it makes your entire body, from the hair on your head to the tip of your toes, stand and applaud.

This is why the dish has survived with its recipe relatively unchanged since the Middle Ages. It's the reason I fell in love with cooking. I was eighteen and living on my own for the first time and emerging from my Chef Boyardee phase—that brief period when everything I made came from a can or the freezer. I wanted to make lasagna. I loved my mother's lasagna almost as much as I could love anything. One afternoon I drove home and my mom handed me the hand-written card that is on my kitchen counter today.

My mother's lasagna had its roots in my Nonnie's kitchen, which meant it really had its roots in Italy, where the ancient Greeks are said to have brought the first recipe to Rome in the second century. Meaning my mom's recipe had been tried and tested for ages. It was her go-to for every special occasion except Thanksgiving and Christmas.

"What should I know about making it?" I asked.

"It's easy," she said. "Come over and watch me the next time I make it."

"Watch me" was the key phrase in her invitation. Lasagna is one of those things you can make off a recipe card, but my mom never followed the recipe exactly. Neither did my Nonnie. The basics are the same, but it's always a pinch of this, a little of that, maybe a little extra of something else. You can take a freeway or drive the blue highways and back roads and end up at relatively the same place, but the experience along the way influences how you feel about the trip.

I still remember the first time I did it on my own in my tiny little house. I took it out of the oven, picked off a bit of one corner, and when I finally tasted a full-size piece, I thought, *Whoa, that's amazing. I can cook.*

Over time, it also became my go-to. Even when *The Silver Palate Cookbook*'s chicken Marbella became the thing everyone made when they wanted to impress family and friends, I still relied on my mom's lasagna. I made it for Ed and Wolfie. I made it for my parents. I made it for my brothers. I proudly announced its arrival fresh from the oven when all of us gathered for special occasions at the beach house. I shared its story to kick off the ninth season of *Valerie's Home Cooking,* an episode that I titled "Honoring Nonnie."

Somewhere along the way, I varied my mom's recipe. Instead of using ricotta cheese the way she did, I substituted Parmesan and a rich béchamel, a white sauce made from a roux and milk. I called my version lasagna *alla besciamella.* My mom called hers lasagna the way it's supposed to be made.

After my first cookbook was published, she called me to say that she found a mistake.

"Where?" I asked.

"The lasagna," she said.

"What's wrong with it?" I asked, concerned about a misprint.

"There's no ricotta," she said.

"Oh, we're going to do this?" I replied.

"I'm sure it's still delicious," she said. "It's just not right."

I laughed. "Okay, you English-Irish woman."

· · · · · · · · ·

Perhaps the only part about lasagna that rivals the burnt corners is taking the leftovers out of the fridge the next day, which is what I do. Next comes the unwinnable debate: Is leftover lasagna better heated up or cold?

For those preferring it warm, I recommend cutting a piece and putting it in the oven at 350 degrees for about twenty minutes; try to avoid a quick hit in the microwave. The wait is worth it. I slice a slender piece, center it attractively on a plate, and eat it cold. It reminds me of a multilayer cake, savory minus the sweet, and it is satisfying in a way that tells me my taste for lasagna the previous day was more about feeding my soul than it was my stomach — the same as it is now.

I have been worrying about Ed. I have also been thinking about how Wolfie is managing, how close he is to Ed, and how that love is like a string he keeps tying in ever tighter and smaller knots in a courageous and unflagging effort to keep a much larger ship from drifting away in a strong current. My son keeps so much inside. Divorce created an invisible wall. Most things with either one of us are on a need-to-know basis. Cancer hasn't changed this.

Sometimes I have to pry the information out of him. I am concerned that he inherited the best of Ed and the worst of me.

Yet sometimes we stare at each other the way family members do, with familiarity and fear and instant understanding, no words necessary. I love my son till it hurts. The way I think he loves his dad and me.

In therapy, people talk about needing a toolbox — different tools for different situations. My mom's recipe box is mine. I go to the recipe box when I need ideas. I also go to it when I need to commune with those who came before me and still hover in that invisible place nearby. It provides reminders and helps me to reset in ways I didn't anticipate when I brought it home after we moved my mom and dad to assisted living. The recipes are written in my mom's beautiful script. Some are as crisp and fresh as the day she wrote them. Others are worn and stained, containing not just recipes but stories; they are three-by-five platters on which memories are brought to the table and deliciously revisited.

Like the lasagna. When I took out the card yesterday, I could hear myself calling her that first time and asking how to make it.

Today, it's another question: How do you get through it? Where is the card for that? Under appetizers? Meat and poultry? Salads? Dessert?

It's not like my mom and I were even that close, not in the way where I called her for advice during troubling times. Then again, maybe I underestimated her — and us. When I was younger, I had lots of questions. What do you put in your meat loaf? What was in Nonnie's red sauce? How do you make your cheesecake? She always told me.

Let's see what she has to say now.

I go rummaging in my toolbox and pull out a card. Onion rings. Bent and discolored by what I assume are blotches of grease and oil, the card appears to have spent a lot of time next to the stove. Except I can't remember her making onion rings that often. The next card I fish out is titled NEW ORLEANS RED BEANS & RICE. She really got into New Orleans–style food after she and my dad moved to Louisiana, and even though I wasn't living at home at the time, I remember her serving these with nearly everything when I visited.

I try one more card.

Now it's like a game. Like I am dealing tarot cards.

Bread.

Huh. Simple white bread. I read the instructions out loud. "Two cups of water, lukewarm; one package or a cake of yeast."

I stop and think. I have big jars of yeast. How much is a package? Usually about two and a quarter teaspoons.

"Three teaspoons of sugar; two teaspoons of salt; and three cups of flour. Heat and add five tablespoons of margarine. Add three more cups of flour, mix and knead for about ten minutes. Put into a greased bowl."

The recipe ends there. I look at the backside of the card, hoping to find the rest of the steps, but it's blank. I see only a smudge, a fingerprint—my mom's.

"How many rises, Mom?" I say. "Do I make a loaf? Or do I turn the dough into little rolls? What's the deal? Where's the rest? It's not like you to leave it unfinished."

Then I get it. She is talking to me as clearly as she did in the past. In the Bible, it's referred to as the staff of life. At the Last Supper, Jesus passed out pieces of unleavened bread, a symbol of his broken body. It provides nourishment to the physical body. It also feeds the soul. It is a gift from God. It can sustain life. It can be shared.

"Take this and eat . . ."

I don't think it was an accident that I pulled out a recipe for bread. Or that the last steps were left for me to figure out on my own.

. . . . . . . . .

The recipes in that little box tell more of a story than I was aware of, from the early days of my parents' marriage when my mom was learning to cook and fighting for acceptance to my first eight years in Delaware and my parents' moves to Michigan, Los Angeles, Oklahoma, and Shreveport. Almost all of my memories of family meals are from when we lived in Delaware. I recall sitting around the kitchen table or, if it was a special occasion, in the dining room, where my mom had painted one entire wall with a beautiful mural of the Italian coast from the perspective of people sitting on a balcony.

I have no idea how she found the time to design and paint such a monumental work while taking care of four small children and preparing three meals a day for a family of six. Plus, she sewed all my clothes, as well as clothes for my Barbie dolls. We moved to Michigan when I was eight; to LA in 1971; and by age fifteen, I was spending most of my time at the studio working on *One Day at a Time*.

A year or two later, someone on the set introduced me to café au lait and I thought my taste level had skyrocketed. At eighteen, I was living on my own and loved to eat out at the Moustache Café, a trendy French bistro on the even trendier Melrose Avenue. I ordered quiche, a dish that struck me as the height of sophistication. I learned to make it on my own and proudly served it to my mom and dad.

*This is quiche.*

*Quiche, meet my parents.*

Then my mom called one day to tell me that she had found a recipe for Famous Amos cookies.

"The actual cookies?" I asked.

"Yes. Famous Amos chocolate chip cookies," she said.

"I need to copy that recipe," I said.

For kicks, I sift through the dessert section of the recipe box and there is the card: FAMOUS AMOS COOKIES.

The day I brought home my mom's recipe box, I also gathered an armful of cookbooks, several dating back to the early fifties and one from 1947. Aside from a bunch of dishware and utensils and pots and pans that I didn't need and decided to donate, I looked long and hard at her pot holders: two oversize gloves that literally had black burn marks on the palm sides. The fabric was paper thin; she had used them for ages, as long as I could remember, until they were unusable.

I put them in the trash. Remembering this helps straighten out my anxiety about Ed and Wolfie. Recipes can be shared. It's an ongoing conversation. The handling of hot dishes, the heavy lifting, the labor itself, I was going to have to do that myself. But I appreciated and accepted any and all help along the way.

· · · · · · · · ·

Which is ironic. For so long, I was afraid to ask for help. In anything. I was under the false presumptions of youth and ignorance that I shouldn't admit I didn't know how to do something. It turns out that asking for help is easy. Years ago, I asked Ed to teach me how to play a particular Patty Griffin song that I liked. I sang a bit of it for him.

"Oh yeah, that's easy," he said, grabbing a guitar—one of the many that always seemed to be within his arm's reach—and strumming the song as if he had played it a hundred times. Then he handed me the guitar and showed me the first and second chords and the up and down rhythm of the strum as he slowly guided my hand.

"Okay, now you try it," he said.

I began the song in fine form but stopped abruptly just a few words in and turned to Ed with a look of helplessness.

"How do you do that chord again?"

"Oh come on, it's easy," he said.

"Easy for you."

I can still picture where the two of us were sitting that night.

· · · · · · · · ·

My mom's recipe box gave me access to her meat loaf, scalloped potatoes, and risotto. It also gave me secrets and stories. It gave me a connection to family history. It reminded me of all the meals that got us through difficult times and helped us enjoy the good times.

It gave me permission to change and tweak ingredients to my own taste. It taught me that cooking has as much to do with feeding our spirits and souls as it does satisfying our hunger—and most of what we hunger for has to do with our spirits and souls.

The last time I made dinner for my parents was in the summer of 2016. We didn't have reason to suspect it at the time, but it would be the last time we would eat together. My dad passed away four or five months later, and my mom was not strong enough to make the trip again. I served lasagna. What else was I going to make? At the table, my mom sat next to me and after taking her first bite, she turned to me, nodding and smiling as she finished chewing.

"This is delicious," she said. "What did you change?"

"Not a thing, Mom," I said. "It's your recipe."

# My Mom's Lasagna

Except for my substituting no-boil noodles (it's a huge time-saver), this is pretty much the lasagna that turned my mom from an English-Irish girl from Jersey into a real Italian cook. Remember to save one of the crispy corners for yourself.

| | |
|---|---|
| 1 | pound lean ground beef |
| ½ | pound hot Italian sausage |
| 1 | small yellow onion, chopped |
| 2 | cloves garlic, minced |
| 1 | teaspoon dried oregano |
| 2 | tablespoons tomato paste |
| 1 | 26.42-ounce container strained tomatoes, such as Pomì |
| 2 | large eggs |
| 30 | ounces part-skim ricotta |

| | |
|---|---|
| 1 | 16-ounce bag shredded mozzarella |
| ⅓ | cup plus ¼ cup grated Parmesan |
| 1 | tablespoon chopped fresh basil |
| 1 | tablespoon chopped fresh oregano |
| ½ | teaspoon kosher salt |
| | Freshly ground black pepper |
| 1 | 1-pound box no-boil lasagna noodles |

*(recipe continued on next page)*

Preheat the oven to 375 degrees F.

Place a large sauté pan over medium-high heat and add the beef and sausage. Cook, stirring occasionally, until it begins to brown, about 2 minutes.

Add the onions, garlic, and dried oregano and cook until the onions are softened and the meat is cooked through, 3 to 4 minutes.

Stir in the tomato paste and cook for 30 seconds, then add the tomatoes and cook until the sauce has thickened slightly, about 5 minutes. Remove from the heat and set aside.

Beat the eggs in a large bowl. Add the ricotta, 1 cup mozzarella, ⅓ cup Parmesan, basil, oregano, salt, and pepper, and stir to combine.

Spread a thin layer of sauce on the bottom of a 9-by-13-inch baking dish.

Arrange a layer of noodles over the sauce and top with a third of the ricotta filling. Spoon over a layer of sauce and top with another layer of noodles. Continue with 2 more layers of ricotta, sauce, and noodles, ending with a top layer of noodles.

Spoon a thin layer of the remaining sauce over the top, sprinkle the remaining mozzarella and Parmesan over the noodles, and cover with aluminum foil.

Bake for 45 minutes, then uncover and cook until the cheese is golden and the lasagna is bubbling, another 15 to 20 minutes.

Let stand for 10 to 15 minutes before serving.

# Learning How to Listen

## SUMMER 2020

WOLFIE CALLS LATE IN the afternoon and says he wants to come by the house to play with Bubba. He arrives with his girlfriend, Andraia, whom I adore, but not as much as Henry—a large, fluffy, white cat who is in love with her—does. He says both of them have had a long, taxing day at their respective jobs and that they want to relax away from their screens.

"Are you going to stay for dinner?" I ask.

"No, we're just going to hang out," he says.

"I'll make something," I say.

"You don't have to," he says.

Two hours later, we are eating dinner. I knew they were going to stay when Wolfie said they were going to hang out. "We're just going to hang out" meant they had nothing planned for later on. Those two words—"hang out"—are code for the rest of the day and night is open. These days, of course, nothing is open and no one is going anywhere, but I knew from Wolfie's tone that he wanted to be home, where his mom would fix dinner and he could snuggle with his cats.

For dinner, since I didn't have much in the refrigerator, I made tuna melts. I mixed the tuna with a couple of hard-boiled eggs, a delicious and underappreciated combination in my opinion, and layered on a few slices of provolone although pepper jack would have been my first choice if I had had any available.

The sandwiches are devoured.

As we eat, I catch up with Andraia, who is brilliant, curious, and fascinating to speak with, though I understand only half of what she says about her work. In addition to occasional modeling jobs, she is a software engineer at one of the large computer companies. I love that she is a young woman who leads with her brain. In college, she majored in computer science after getting the programming bug as a young girl. At ten years old, she tells me, she wanted to make a Backstreet Boys website and she read the page code.

"You read the page code and just understood it?" I ask.

"Yes," she says.

"I love it," I say. "I don't even know where to find the page code."

Wolfie is quiet and content to listen to Andraia and me chat until I mention spending the weekend at our beach house. With an impish smile, he leans forward and says he might go on eBay and look for replacements for the computer games he lost in what is known in our house as the "flood." The flood happened almost fifteen years ago. A leak in my bathroom dripped into the playroom directly beneath it and ruined Wolfie's collection of computer games. They had to be thrown out. I am amused by his enduring distress and laugh.

"It's not funny," he says. "Those were sacred games."

I look at him with raised eyebrows. "Sacred?"

"I had a Sega Genesis. Also a Saturn console, which was rare. And a Sega Pico, which was this kids' learning center that was really cool. And more. Everything got destroyed."

"Sorry," I say, then I cringe as I picture that scene.

"How come the flood got so bad?" Andraia asks.

"I didn't hear the drip," I say.

Now it is Wolfie's turn to look at me with raised eyebrows. "For three years?"

· · · · · · · · ·

I will neither confirm nor deny.

My problem is not whether I can hear. It's what I hear and what I don't hear. For much of my life, I have only heard the criticism I levied against myself when I looked in the mirror. I confirmed it when I got on the scale. The details changed, as did the number on the scale, but the message was always the same: you need fixing. Which I translated as "you need to lose ten pounds."

I was telling myself other things, like *Go see Mom and Dad* and *Follow your passion* and later *Check in on Ed*, and I was fortunate to have heard those things. But so many other things were drowned out by *You need to lose ten pounds.* And the truth was that those ten pounds or whatever number happened to come up that day represented all the other issues and insecurities I wasn't tending to.

Here's the deal. When you carry around a heavy bag of emotions and don't deal with them, you eventually become that heavy bag. Likewise, when all you tell yourself is that you are fat and have to lose weight, you never hear other people say that you are nice, funny, smart, generous, and kind—all the things that make a person truly beautiful.

It was there. I just couldn't hear it. That you-got-to-lose-ten-pounds voice made me tone deaf to everything else. Not only couldn't I hear myself think, but I also couldn't hear anything or *anyone* else, including all the people who came up to me over the years and said such nice things about me. Imagine such a blessing and not being able to hear it. Like missing Mozart. Or a bottle of champagne popping and baby's laughter.

For me, it was easier and more believable to hear the negative. The voices in my head confirmed everything I said to myself when I missed the number on the scale even when the facts and the entire world said otherwise.

I missed out on so much. One night shortly after Ed and I were married, I was jerked awake from a deep sleep by noise—music being played over and over again outside the bedroom door. I was annoyed. I didn't even hear the catchy melody. Instead, the voice in my head said, *He has to do that now? When I have to get up early in the morning for work?*

I tried rolling over and shutting my eyes tighter. I put the pillow over my head. I could still hear the music—*ba-ba . . . ba-ba-ba-ba*. Finally, I got up, walked across the dark room, and opened the door, where I found my husband sitting on the floor in front of his mini synthesizer, a knot of elbows and knees and long brown hair hovering over a keyboard.

He looked up at me with a sheepish grin. Our cat Edgar was snuggled in his lap. Edgar looked up at me, too. Both of them knew I was pissed.

"Sorry," Ed said.

"You have to do that here?" I asked. "Right outside the bedroom door?"

He shrugged. Like he couldn't help it.

"Please stop," I said as lovingly as possible. "I beg you to stop. I have to get up at five in the morning."

As I shut the door and got back into bed, I heard Ed say, "Love you," then the music started back up again, though only for a minute or so as he eventually got up from the floor and worked the rest of the night in his music room down the hall.

It was a good thing that Ed didn't listen to me. That song is now instantly recognizable as "Jump." It came out on the band's *1984* album and was Van Halen's first and only number one song. We have laughed about this for years.

. . . . . . . . .

I began learning how to listen when I first heard the music Wolfie was writing. It was the summer of 2015, and Wolfie was on tour with Van Halen. This was his third and final tour with the band. Eager to visit him, I met up with them back East, and one afternoon Wolfie asked if I wanted to hear something he was working on. He was casual about it. He didn't say he was writing songs. He didn't describe it as new music of his own. He said it was "some stuff I'm working on."

He was humble, uncertain, and guarded, which is normal for him, but as an expert in Wolfie-speak, I knew that, in addition to rehearsals, video games, and his girlfriend, this "stuff" must be important to him.

"They're rough, not even fully developed demos," he cautioned, as we settled into the back of the tour bus.

I was speechless after the first song, which he had titled "Epiphany." Halfway through the second song, "Resolve," I was trying to keep it together and not doing a very good job of it. The back of my throat was swollen and achy and ready to burst, because that's where I was stuffing all the emotion.

"One more?" he asked.

I nodded.

That's when the dam burst. The third song was titled "Distance," a slow, moody ballad that began with a simple drumbeat and a guitar strum. After the song continued like that for a few seconds, I heard Wolfie's voice. He was humming. I looked over at him. He was watching me for a reaction.

"I don't have the words yet," he said.

"I still almost hear them," I said, shutting my eyes and letting the music into me. "It's like I can almost hear the words."

And then I did. The chorus kicked in and I heard Wolfie singing.

*No matter what the distance is, I will be with you*
*No matter what the distance is, you'll be okay*

Without attempting to wipe the tears from my eyes, I hugged Wolfie and listened to the rest of the track with him in my arms. At the time, we did not know that Ed was going to get so sick. We were still three years from hearing that the cancer had spread. But Wolfie, having toured and recorded with Van Halen since 2007, had already been through a lot with his dad, and whether or not he knew it, he was preparing himself for the next inevitable stage, and he was doing a much better job of it than I was. I could not have been prouder.

When I saw Ed backstage at the arena later that day, I literally pulled him away from wherever he was headed to and asked if he had heard Wolfie's music.

"Yeah," he said.

"Can you believe it?" I said.

His eyes lit up in the way they did whenever he talked about Wolfie, and he wiped away a tear.

"I know," he said. "He's amazing."

· · · · · · · · ·

Even in the early, raw, unfinished state of Wolfie's music, I heard so much of what we had talked about over the years, what Wolfie and his dad had talked about, what the three of us had discussed when we got together, and what all of us individually had thought or were thinking and were too frightened to say. I heard Wolfie's talent and his emotions, his sensitivity and his passion, and . . . his love.

"How do you do it?" I asked.

"Like Dad," he said. "I listen for the music."

When Wolfie was a little boy, I would take him out on the Van Halen tour every so often so he could spend time with his dad, and Ed would bring him onstage for a father-son duet. I think it was Ed's favorite part of the show, and Wolfie loved it — the novelty, the crowd, and, most of all, making his dad happy. I prayed he wouldn't go into music. It was and is such a rough business. People are so judgmental. And with his last name, everything was going to be even harder. Every note he played would be compared to his dad's music.

As he got older, I resigned myself to the fact that he didn't have a choice. Besides an abundance of natural talent, Wolfie also had the gift of hearing music in his head or in the air or wherever those ideas come from. Ed gave him permission not only to listen to it but also to follow it. He encouraged him to play and write. Ed was aware of the influence music could have on people through its ability to convey emotions — happiness, sadness, joy, excitement, the thrill of being alive in the moment. He knew it could change lives. It had changed his.

I don't think anything changed Ed's life more than playing alongside Wolfie on three Van Halen tours. That is until he heard Wolfie's own music.

Listening made me feel the same way. But Wolfie didn't let me hear the demos of his songs again until 2018. This time they had lyrics. Though they were still being produced, they were more polished and put together. Wolfie wrote all the songs, both the music and the words, and he played every instrument. I was so deeply moved after hearing what he was able to express in those songs—thoughts about love, depression, regret—that I sat and stared at him, shaking my head in awe.

Later that night, I sent him a text praising everything he had done as a musician, sharing the concerns I had always had about his going into music, but finally explaining that it was his gifts as a songwriter that had helped me to understand the depths of his artistry and that, even more important, those songs had given me insight into him as a young man and I loved what I heard.

"Thank you for letting me listen," I said. "I love you."

. . . . . . . . .

Wolfie was ready to release his album in 2018 and go on tour, but after Ed learned his cancer had spread, he put everything on hold to spend time with his dad. He used the time to tinker and fine-tune, and every so often I heard an updated version of one of his songs. One day he mentioned that Ed's favorite was "Think It Over." I was jealous. I wanted a copy of the songs for myself so I could listen often enough to have my own favorite.

I didn't really need to have a favorite. But as his proud mama, I did need a copy of those songs. All of them.

"Fine," he said. "The next time you come over to my house, I'll upload them onto your phone."

I went over to Wolfie's house the same day Ed showed up and all of us shared the spinach and crab dip I had left over from *The Kelly Clarkson Show*. I got there first and gave Wolfie my phone while I prepared the dip and arranged the crackers and crudités on a plate. I was eager to get his music downloaded. He was excited for me to sit down and listen to his songs. But he had an unexpected change of heart about putting them on my phone.

"Can you just listen to them here?" he said. "You can come over whenever you want."

"It's just for me," I said. "I've been asking for months."

"But—"

"I promise I won't play them for anyone." I started to cry.

"Oh my God, Mom," he said. "I didn't think you'd be like this." He walked across the kitchen and hugged me.

"I'll give you the songs," he said.

When Ed opened the front door and walked into the house, Wolfie had finished downloading all the songs and was showing me where on my phone I could find them. At my request, he was also playing his album on his home speakers. The music was loud, the way our family likes our rock and roll. Ed cocked his head to the side and listened. His eyes sparkled with pride. His smile was even brighter. I looked up from my phone and matched his grin.

"Hiya," I said. "He just downloaded his songs onto my phone."

"Nice," he said, with an approving nod.

Then he spotted the bowl of spinach and crab dip and the crackers on the table, and said, "Hey, what's that?"

"It's delicious," I said.

· · · · · · · · ·

Months after Ed and I talked in George Lopez's car on Thanksgiving, I thought of an Italian proverb that said from listening comes wisdom and from speaking, repentance. That explained the way I felt about that conversation. When Ed shared the kinship and closeness he still had for me, and the love he still felt, adding that he hoped it didn't sound weird or awkward, it had more of an impact on me than I knew at the time. I felt good about the things I was able to tell him, too, and after we went back inside, I thought that was it, conversation finished, feelings shared, all good. But I kept thinking about it, and still do.

It allowed me to see that our twenty-year marriage didn't fail as much as it evolved into a friendship, then into a different form of love. I already knew this. But hearing it from Ed felt good in the moment and even better as time went on.

The next time I saw Ed was in the hospital. It was January 2020 and he was recovering from a procedure on his back. When I walked into his room, he was in his underwear, brushing his teeth. He looked pretty good for someone who had cancer in his lungs and brain and wherever else it had spread. A large white bandage covered the spot on his back where he had had surgery a few days earlier. He was bobbing his head to Wolfie's music, which was playing on a couple of Ed's speakers at a volume atypical for hospitals.

"Pretty good," I said.

"It's fucking amazing," he said.

. . . . . . . . .

Now, six months later, life has changed. We are locked down in our homes, we see only those in our pods, and we wear masks if we go outside. I am being told that we might tape *Kids Baking Championship* later this summer. Ordinarily, that would trigger panic followed by a diet followed by anxiety. But my own work—and my work with Angie—is helping me to manage those voices in my head that are always telling me to lose ten pounds, be better, and fix myself.

I hear those voices, I acknowledge them, I try to figure out what they want, then I put them in the Trash Room, the Past Room, or some other storage bin. In their place, I hear different voices, more positive voices, kinder and more loving voices. It has an effect. The worries and insecurities I would typically have about being in front of the camera get put in their place, and I am able to focus on how much fun it will be to hang out with my friend Duff and laugh with all the remarkable kid bakers on the show.

Ditto with my own kid. When Wolfie updates me about Ed, I am not filtering the information through my own mental cacophony. Instead, I am present for him and more able to understand that he speaks in code, telling me what he thinks I need to know about Ed and also what he needs me to know as his mom. The two are not the same thing. It is amazing what I can hear with a clear head. It's like driving with a clean windshield.

I only wish I had been able to do this sooner. I think about the arguments I had with my mother and that one showdown at the beach house years ago. When she asked why I didn't want to talk and be closer, I think what she really meant was why won't you open up to me and let me open up to you. I couldn't — not with her. There was just too much gunk. Just because she was ready to open up didn't mean I was ready. I didn't have that skill set — not yet.

I wish it had been otherwise. I see other mothers and daughters with tight relationships, and I wonder how my life and my mom's life would have been different if we'd been that way, too. We were so alike in so many ways. She ate her emotions. She was always on a diet. She didn't fully come into her own until later in life. It makes me sad for what could have been, but maybe it's just the way it was supposed to be.

It took Ed and me until this past Thanksgiving to talk and hear what was really in each other's hearts. I wish we had done that ten years earlier. It is a bright, shiny moment amid what is turning out to be a truly weird and terrible year. But Ed and I trade texts. Even though this damn Covid has me nervous about going to see him, I promise to drop by, that is if I ever go anyplace but the grocery store.

Strangely enough, I have been hearing the intro to Van Halen's song "Women in Love" in my head. Though Ed wrote it before we met, the intro has been a favorite of mine since I first heard it. Backstage at shows, while he was tuning his guitars and warming up his fingers, I always asked him to play it. I didn't have to say anything more than "Please play it," and he knew exactly what I wanted to hear. Occasionally, he snuck it into one of his solos and turned to me on the side of the stage with a playful glint in his eyes to see if I was listening.

I am determined to make more good memories by listening to the good stuff. To that end, the best advice comes from my kid. One day I ask Wolfie about writing the lyrics to his songs. I am impressed by the sensitivity and depth of the subjects he has tackled. When I was his age, I struggled to express my emotions. Just getting a handle on them was a challenge. Even now, at my age, I am still learning. Wolfie explains that melody comes before words, but while he is writing, he is coming up with what he calls mouth shapes—"Words and phrases that feel good in my mouth," he tells me.

"Instead of trying to shoehorn a bunch of words into a song because I've written them down in my notebook, I listen for words that sound good and feel good."

"You listen for a feel?" I ask.

"You can hear when something sounds right."

I get it. And that's how I finally learned how to listen.

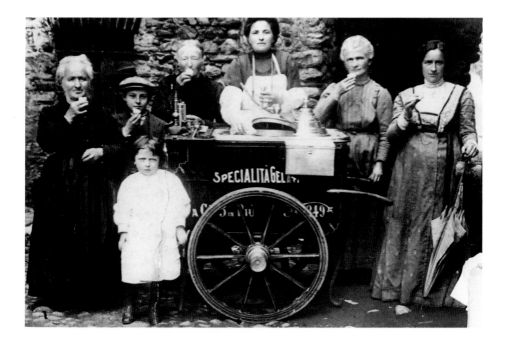

Three generations — my great-great-grandmother, my great-grandmother, and my grandmother — with Maria's gelato cart in Lanzo Torinese outside of Turin, Italy.

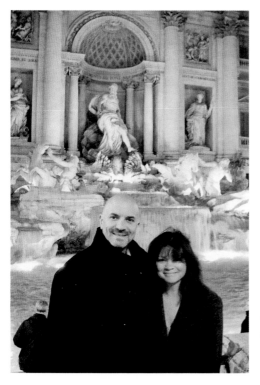

Tom and I finally finding the Trevi Fountain after arriving in Rome very jet-lagged.

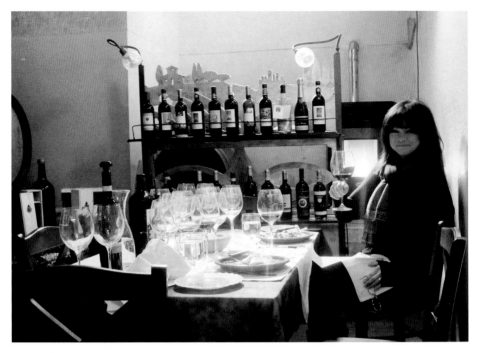

The little winery in Tuscany where I had lasagna for the first time with béchamel sauce. My mother never forgave me for changing her recipe.

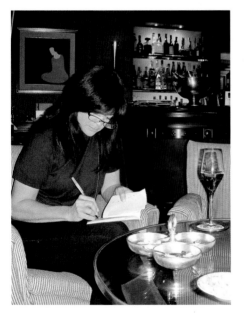

Journaling in the Hotel Eden bar in Rome. Every entry says, "I love it here."

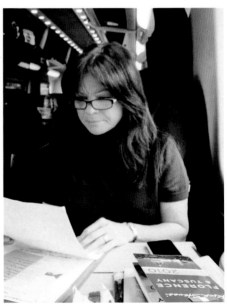

On the train to Florence, researching where we are going to dine.

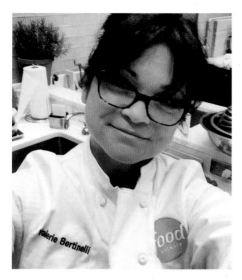

In the Food Network kitchens with my first official chef's coat that my producer, Mary Beth, gave me.

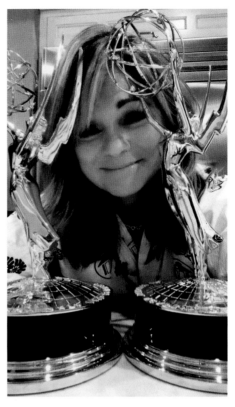

The two Emmys I was fortunate enough to win in 2019. Come and get me, Imposter Syndrome.

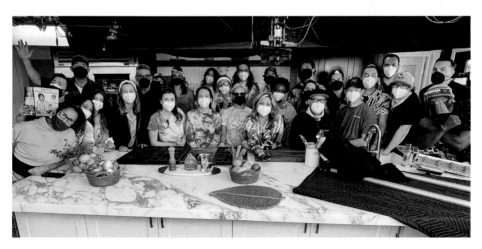

My happy place — shooting *Valerie's Home Cooking* with this amazing crew.

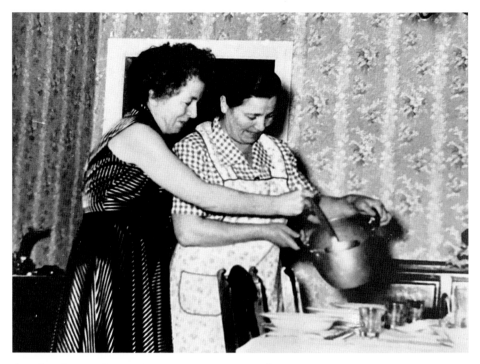

Angelina Bertinelli and Maria Francesca Possio Crosa — my grandmother and great-grandmother.

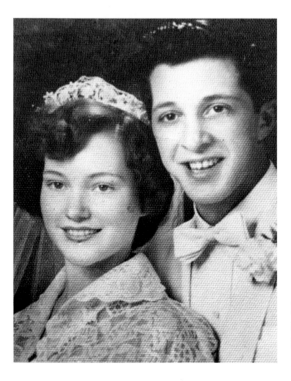

My parents — my mom is seventeen and my dad is twenty. Crazy.

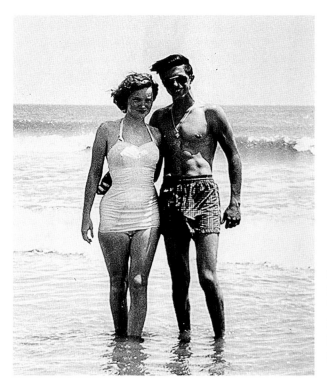

My parents on their
honeymoon in 1954.
They look gorgeous.
My mom was a stunner
but never believed it.
Sound familiar?

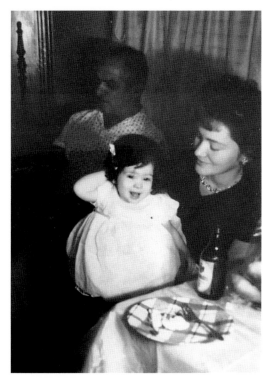

My beautiful mom holding me.
This is one of the few pictures I have
of Nazzareno Bertinelli, my grand-
father, who is in the background.

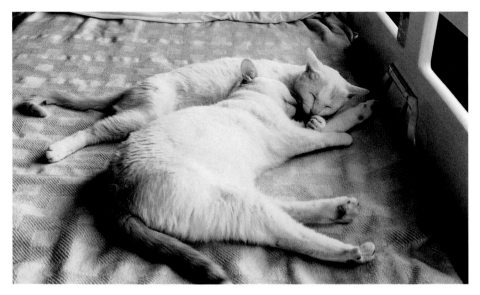

Bubba and Beau together again on my dad's bed the day after we found Bubba.

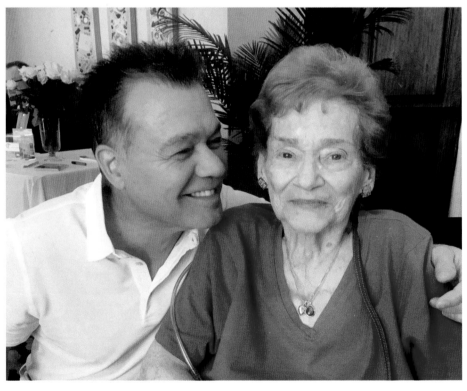

The picture Ed texted me after my mother passed. You can see how much he adored her.

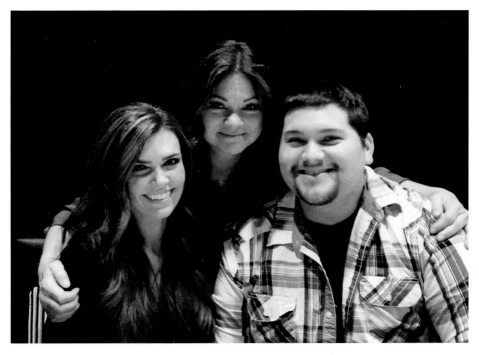

Wolfie, Andraia, and I celebrating at a joint twenty-fifth birthday party for them.

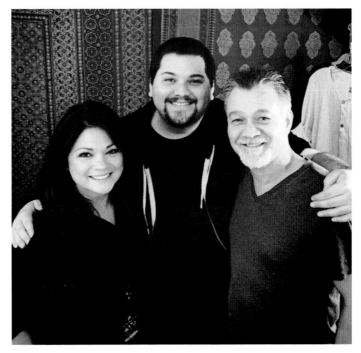

Backstage in Ed's dressing room on the road in 2015.

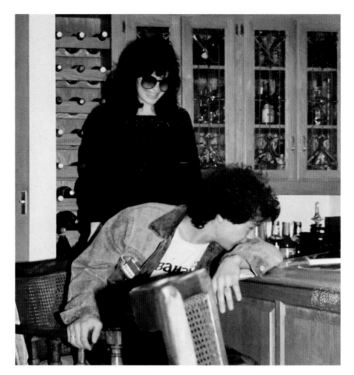

Ed's surprise thirtieth birthday party that we were three hours late for.

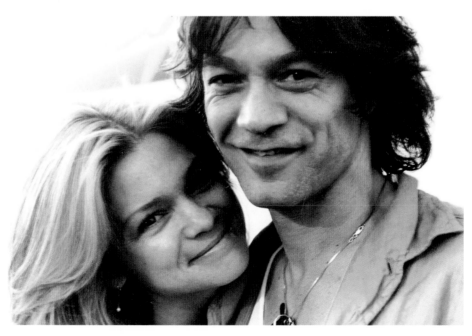

This is later in our marriage, and those are the sober eyes of two people who love each other and will always love each other.

# Tuna Egg Salad Melts

I recommend playing Wolfie's album while you are making this sandwich. Then you get two of my favorites at the same time.

| | | | |
|---|---|---|---|
| 2 | 5-ounce cans albacore tuna, drained well | ½ | cup mayonnaise |
| 4 | hard-boiled eggs, chopped | 1 | tablespoon Dijon mustard |
| 1 | celery stalk, chopped (about ⅓ cup) | ½ | teaspoon smoked paprika |
| ⅓ | cup chopped dill pickles or relish | 3 | to 4 tablespoons unsalted butter, room temperature |
| ¼ | cup chopped Tamed jalapeños | 8 | slices sourdough bread |
| 3 | scallions, trimmed and roughly chopped | 8 | slices pepper jack cheese or cheese of your choice |
| | | | Kosher salt |
| | | | Freshly ground black pepper |

Add the tuna, chopped eggs, celery, dill pickles, jalapeños, and scallions to a mixing bowl. Mix to incorporate and break up any large chunks of tuna.

*(recipe continued on next page)*

To the tuna mixture, add the mayonnaise, mustard, and smoked paprika. Use a rubber spatula to mix until evenly combined. Set aside.

Arrange the sliced bread on a clean work surface. Butter one side of each piece of bread. Flip the bread over so it is now butter-side down. Place 1 piece of cheese on 4 of the slices of bread, tearing in half if needed to fit the bread comfortably. Divide the tuna mixture evenly over the cheese. Top with the remaining 4 slices of cheese, tearing if necessary, and top with the remaining bread, butter-side up.

Heat a large pan over medium heat. Once the pan is warm, add 2 to 3 sandwiches or as many as your pan will allow without over-crowding it. Cook until golden brown and crisp, 3 to 4 minutes. Flip the sandwiches and cook for an additional 2 to 3 minutes until golden brown and the cheese is melted.

Transfer the sandwiches to a cutting board and continue cooking the remaining sandwiches.

Slice in half and serve immediately.

# I Don't Know How Much
# Longer We Have

## OCTOBER 2020

ONE DAY THERE IS something in Wolfie's voice. Whether it is a change in his tone, a catch in his throat, or just my mother's intuition, I hear it.

I don't mention anything at first. I don't want to, and I don't know what to say.

I have a habit of blurting out whatever is on my mind, sometimes for the better and sometimes not, and this is one of those times when I don't want to blow it. So I err on the side of biting my tongue.

A short time later, Wolfie calls me from outside Ed's room at Saint John's Hospital in Santa Monica.

"I don't know how much longer we have," he says.

My brother Patrick had said those exact same words to me about my mother. She lived another six months after he sounded that alarm.

This is a different situation. I know it. I hear it in Wolfie's voice. He wouldn't be telling me this if it wasn't true—and it's probably more dire than he lets on.

"Okay, I'll be there," I say.

Though Covid has complicated matters and robbed us of precious time together, being there for each other, one way or another, is what our lives have been about for much of the year. A few weeks earlier, Wolfie walked out of Ed's hospital room looking for me. When I saw him in the hall, the look in his eyes said everything. I instinctively reached out and he crumbled into my arms. My six-foot little boy. I hugged him as tightly as I could. I don't know where maternal strength comes from, but I was full of it and wanted to give him all of it.

"I'm sorry you're going through this," I said. "I'm sorry your dad is going through this. I'm sorry for all of us."

Wolfie, his head buried in my shoulder, nodded.

"You've been so strong for so long," I said. "You're allowed to not be strong. You don't have to be strong anymore."

· · · · · · · · ·

I make a promise to myself to be at the hospital every day. I feel unprepared, like this has snuck up on me. I can still hear Ed two years ago at Wolfie's rehearsal casually mentioning that he has just been diagnosed with brain cancer. He was so nonchalant about it, like he was telling me about his latest new car. Later, I found out he had stage IV lung cancer, though I don't recall Ed or Wolfie actually telling me the cancer had spread there, too. If they did, it didn't register, which seems unlikely. I can't believe I would hear "stage IV" and not get freaked out.

But I have watched Ed deal with cancer for twenty years. He has always said he was going to beat it, and I believed him. Each time it popped up, he swatted it away with the newest drugs and treatments. Ed beats everything. He gets stopped for drunk driving and they don't take him to jail or even write him up. Why? Because he's Eddie Van Halen. His talent has created a magic-carpet ride through life.

Not that he didn't have hard times. His childhood was painful. When his parents moved from Indonesia to the Netherlands, Ed and Alex were subjected to racist slurs and teased as half-breeds because of their parents' mixed ethnicity. After moving to Pasadena, they were extremely poor. They shared a house with other families. His mother worked as a maid, his dad as a janitor. Ed had tears in his eyes as he told me about their fake Christmas presents — boxes that were wrapped but empty, so when people came over to their house, they would think the Van Halens were just like any other family.

He had such a big sensitive heart and was a gentle old soul. It killed him that he hurt people. He was tortured knowing he had hurt me and disappointed his son in the past. In my 2008 book *Losing It*, I wrote to Ed in the acknowledgments: "You're a good man, believe it. When you do, you'll be free." I didn't want him to feel guilty anymore about things that had happened in the past. I had forgiven him. I wanted him to forgive himself.

When he finally got sober five years ago, he was able to let go and discover that he really was that good, kindhearted man I had described, and I think he thoroughly enjoyed taking a step back, exhaling, and knowing that he didn't have anything more to prove to anyone, especially himself. He was free.

But definitely not finished. In mid-March, Ed had recovered from his back surgery and was set to return to Germany for more cancer treatments. My brother Patrick was going with him. Then Covid hit, flights to Europe were cancelled, and like the rest of us, Ed sheltered at home. We texted and FaceTimed over the summer. Between doctor appointments, he spent most of his time on his sofa watching TV. I wasn't able to see the way his health was declining or how rapidly that was happening, and Ed didn't mention anything to me when we spoke.

I wish I had asked more questions.

I wish I had called more often.

I wish I had just dropped by his house with dinner. *Hey, what-cha doin'? Mind if I hang out on the sofa with you for a while?*

I didn't think it was any of my business.

The damn Covid. It was our Berlin Wall, the electrified fence in *The Hunger Games*, the sonar fence in *Lost*. It kept us from the everyday things that make life rich and meaningful — human contact, touch, kindness. I was reminded of being on a diet. The more we were deprived of these things, the more we craved them.

Neither Ed nor I ever had any thoughts of getting back together. But I always knew he had my back and he knew that I had his.

"Thinking of you," I text him, along with a cat-hugging GIF.

No response.

A few days later . . .

"Morning, just checking in to see how you're feeling," I text.

"Terrible," he responds. "I have a lump on my neck. Cancer sucks."

"I'm sorry."

"How are you? ❤❤❤"

"I think of you every day."

"Thanks. This sucks."

· · · · · · · · ·

August 29, I text Ed: "40 years ago you were playing Shreveport, LA, and my life changed forever. ❤ I hope you're doing well and feeling well."

"40 years!!! That's insane!! Changed mine too!!! Love you Val, hope you're good."

· · · · · · · · ·

In September, Ed suffered a minor stroke. He was already in the hospital, so he received immediate medical care, which was the lone bright spot in a sky that was rapidly filling with dark clouds.

None of us were ready to concede the fight with cancer, but it was proving to be a relentless, tireless, and uncaring opponent. I felt hope dwindle, and though I did not want to admit it, and I kept these terrible feelings to myself, I began to let go of the expectation that there would always be a tomorrow. *See you tomorrow. Talk to you tomorrow. Let's get together next weekend. We should plan a dinner.*

I focused all my energy instead on the present. I did not want to waste a moment. If I wasn't with Ed, I was texting with Wolfie.

Our conversations were reduced to single key words.

*Good.*

*Awake.*

*Comfortable.*

*Sleeping.*

One day Ed struggles to say something. It's afternoon, and Wolfie and I and the rest of the crew are with him. Ed has tried to speak several times since the stroke and we have not been able to understand him. This time, after several tries, Wolfie pulls Ed's oxygen mask off, and asks, "What do you need?"

Ed smiles — his eyes focused and fixed on Wolfie's — and with perfect clarity, he says, "Pizza, please."

The room fills with laughter. Ed's eyes shine. I don't know whether he has cracked a joke or is hungry and wants a slice of pepperoni — one more for the road. He loves pizza. Either way, it warms my heart to know he is still with us.

· · · · · · · · ·

Just after Wolfie informs me that time is running out, Ed's doctor comes into his hospital room. Looking directly at Ed but making sure to also connect with Wolfie, he says there isn't much more they can do for Ed. But if Ed wants, they can continue to try to fight. Without a moment's delay, Ed manages to say, "Let's keep fighting."

For the next week and a half, Wolfie and I are together in Ed's hospital room every day. We sit on either side of him and share stories, make sure he is comfortable, and tell him that we love him. Wolfie has one hand and I have the other. We try not to leave him alone, so if one or both of us aren't there, Ed's brother takes the shift. Janie is also there. Ed knows he is surrounded by the people closest to him and that he is extremely loved.

Wolfie and Ed share earbuds and listen to Wolfie's album together. They have shared music since Wolfie was in diapers and Ed sat him on his lap while he played the piano or the guitar. Ed brightens when he hears "Think It Over," his favorite track. It is the most pop-sounding song on the album; the lyrics are about regret and looking back on past mistakes. By this time, though, Ed has clearly thought things over, made his peace, and all that matters to him is being with his son. As they listen, they hold hands and savor every second they have with each other, just like they used to, just like always.

I spend Friday night sitting on the bed next to Ed. For a while, it is just the two of us. I hold his hand. I stroke his forehead. I smile into his eyes.

"Maybe next time, right?" I say.

Both of us are crying.

"Maybe next time we'll get it right."

· · · · · · · · ·

We are like any other family in this situation. Time doesn't stop as much as it ceases to matter. We know the sand in the hourglass is running low, and we don't look. Our focus is the now. People talk about living in the moment. Nothing puts you in the moment and makes you appreciate what it means to live like watching someone you love die. It's all I think about as I sit there. This is what matters. Love.

In the end, all the other stuff disappears. What's left is love.

Only love is real.

The end comes in slow motion. On Saturday, we spend hours with him, taking turns holding his hands, stroking his arm, smiling into his eyes, and repeating the only thing that matters, "I love you." We make sure that he is comfortable. I feel my heart breaking and wonder how that can be when it is so full of love. Maybe it is too full and threatening to burst.

At night, Ed keeps looking off into the corner. He sees someone, and it seems as if he hears them, too. His face is light, calm, interested, and attentive. I see him smile. It is clear to me that someone is welcoming him, assuring him that he is going to be okay, giving him peace, and I want to know who is there.

But another part of me doesn't want to acknowledge that this is happening. We are still fighting, still hoping. Then Ed lets us know that he is very tired. Wolfie and I get up and gather our stuff. I kiss Ed's forehead.

"Sleep well," I say.

"I'm so tired, I just can't sleep," he says.

"Try," I say. "I love you. I'll see you tomorrow."

"I love you, too," he says.

He says the same thing to Wolfie. "I love you."

Later that night, after all of us have left, Ed suffers another stroke. When Alex shows up in the morning, he can't wake Ed.

He calls Wolfie, and says, "I've been trying to wake your dad for a half hour and haven't been able to." Wolfie calls me, and we race to the hospital. We get to his room a few minutes before Ed is wheeled back in after being given a brain scan. His doctor follows and shows us the scans. We can see the damage without needing an explanation. It is devastating.

"Listen, I know we said we were going to fight, and Ed wanted to fight, but I don't know if we can ever get him awake again," the doctor says. "What we can do, though, is make him really comfortable."

And that's what they do.

· · · · · · · · ·

He hangs on through Monday. On Tuesday morning Wolfie calls and tells me that Ed's breathing has changed and that I have to get to the hospital ASAP.

Defying speed limits, I race across the city, making the thirty-minute drive in half the time. At the hospital, though, I can't find a parking space. A typical LA problem. I am on the phone with Wolfie, who is telling me to hurry. I spot a man walking to his car. *Score!* But he is followed by a very pregnant wife and a toddler who does not cooperate as they try to put him in his car seat. I have been there, but can't they hurry?

"It's taking them forever," I tell Wolfie.

After five minutes (it felt like an hour), I finally pull into the spot and sprint into the hospital. I forget to look if I need to feed a meter or am in a ten-minute zone. I don't care. Let them ticket me or tow the car. Inside the hospital, I stop at the lobby desk and go through the Covid routine I know too well. My temperature is taken; I am handed a new mask; I have to wait for a pass.

"Please hurry," I say. "He's dying."

Because they've seen people dealing with this before, the hospital staff understands why I am in a panic and apologizes. I run across the lobby and catch the first elevator to open. I push the fourth-floor button. At the last second, a woman steps in and pushes two. My patience has never been taxed more. The extra few seconds seem like an eternity. *Why couldn't she have taken the stairs?* I think. *Why didn't I sprint up the stairs? It's a lesson,* I tell myself. Right? It's a lesson. When I finally get to Ed's room, Wolfie is holding his hand. Alex is at the foot of the bed with his son, Malcolm. I pull up a chair and hold Ed's other hand. At some point, Alex's other son, Aric, arrives. So does Janie.

I can see the change in Ed. I have a sense that he has waited for all of us. We tell him that we love him.

"I love you" are the last words Ed says to Wolfie and me, and they are the last words we say to him before he stops breathing. Soon after, a doctor comes in, takes his pulse, and calls the time of death. It's a little after ten o'clock in the morning.

After the doctor leaves the room, none of us moves or speaks. The weight of the moment leaves all of us still, frozen in time, motionless. After about twenty minutes, Janie says she wants to be with her family and leaves. The rest of us stay. I lose track of time until the door opens. A chaplain peeks in and asks if we would like some rosaries. She returns a few moments later, hands out the rosaries, and says a blessing. More time passes. None of us has a desire to leave Ed. Not now. Not ever. We are family. We tell stories about Ed and the Van Halen family. Alex remembers Indonesian words that used to make them laugh as kids. We share stories about Ed's sense of humor. Suddenly, all of us are cracking up. It's bizarre. I would never have imagined sitting in that hospital room hours after Ed has died and laughing as hard or as much, but that is what happens. We laugh — and it is so much better than crying, which we also do a fair amount of the time.

At some point, someone asks if anyone feels like pizza.

"I think Ed would want that," Alex says.

Everyone agrees. Grinning, Alex takes out his cell phone and orders three large pepperoni from a local pizza restaurant. It seems so weird and so right and so Ed.

· · · · · · · · ·

I am numb. In the middle of the night, I wake up sick to my stomach and run to the bathroom. I feel like I am regurgitating the whole year. I haven't thrown up in decades. I go back to bed and sleep late into the morning. Late that afternoon, I drive to Wolfie's house and make him and Andraia dinner—franks and beans, a childhood favorite. Comfort food.

Patrick comes over to offer support. After dinner, we look through several family photo albums that I brought over. My dad put them together years ago. Prompted by the pictures, we trade memories and stories as if we were playing cards and trying to top one another with more tears and more laughter. Where is Ed? Why is he missing this? Maybe he isn't. We can feel him in the room. It inspires Wolfie.

"Ma, I want to finish 'Distance' and release it for Dad," he says.

"That's perfect," I say, then I start to cry. I can't help it. The tears gush out of me. "It's really perfect."

A few days later, Patrick and I are at Wolfie's house again, watching old family Super 8 movies that he and our friend Dave had converted a while back into DVDs. There's one of the three of us —Ed, Wolfie, and I—at the beach when Wolfie was about three years old. It is pure joy. We watch it over and over. Faith Ford was the one who took that video, I recall; then, as we are rewatching it, Faith calls from her home in Louisiana to express her condolences.

"Are you kidding me?" Wolfie says when I tell him who is on the phone.

"I know, right?" I say.

Now I am sure Ed is there with us.

I don't remember how we go from watching these videos and looking at family photos to talking about how these should be compiled and edited into the video for "Distance," but all of us agree that there is no more fitting way to illustrate Wolfie's beautiful song. Ed's music touched so many people and was and remains such an important part of their lives that it feels right to share this very personal part of his and our lives with Wolfie's song.

We talk about it and agree that it can serve as a reminder that love is the best part of us and that we should cherish it.

I know my heart is full of love as we watch these videos.

It is floating on an ocean of tears.

It is full.

And it is afloat.

My thoughts keep going back to Ed in the hospital room, as if I am trying to understand and process what happened even though I know what did. But I do have a new insight. As I sat there holding Ed's hand, crying as he left his physical body, the love we shared stayed with me, and still does, and always will.

Wolfie decides to not only release "Distance" but also include the song on his album. "Now it feels right," he says.

He plays it for us and we cry.

*A life without you, I'm not ready to move on*
*No matter what the distance is I will be with you*
*No matter what the distance is you'll be okay*

# Scrolling Happy

## NOVEMBER 2020

I WAKE UP GROGGY THIS morning. To me, groggy is when I am out of bed and my eyes are open but I feel half-asleep. I still can't see clearly. I need to walk with my arms extended and hands out, feeling the wall and holding on to the banister for dear life as if I were finding my way in the dark. Even the first cup of coffee doesn't lift the fog immediately.

This is different than grumpy. Grumpy is when I turn on cable news while reading the newspaper and start drowning in a pool of disappointment and anger. What is so hard about helping people who need help?

We have a bunch of well-paid people with free lifetime health insurance causing more problems than they solve. Most of them are old men protecting the interests of corporations and their own personal power while talking about making America great as they obscure the facts and turn history into fiction. What does that mean — making America great?

To me, greatness recognizes the powerless and the poor. Greatness works for equity and against injustice. Greatness offers a helping hand and an open heart. Greatness inspires acts of hope, cour-age, and humanity.

But don't get me started. Not while I am groggy.

Here is the rest of my morning.

Coffee.

Cats.

Dog walk.

Crossword.

Silence.

A nice, long, satisfying stretch in the sun.

There, that is better.

In the wake of Ed's death, I am finding my way and working through the grogginess of grief. Wolfie's song "Distance" goes to number one. Emotional triggers are heightened. I allow myself time and space. Words flash in my brain like signs on the highway: *Exhale. Grace. Patience. Breathe. Baby Steps. Laughter. Gratitude.*

On the morning "Distance" is released, Wolfie is interviewed by Howard Stern, who is one of the best if not the best interviewer in the media as long as you aren't the one he's interrogating, as I found out years ago when he focused on my rear end until I basi-cally screamed at him to stop.

With Wolfie, he is respectful, sensitive, and supportive. My fa-vorite part of their conversation is when Wolfie shows Howard the first guitar his dad gave him and confirms that Ed was the world's worst guitar teacher. As Wolfie laughingly recalls, Ed would show him a riff, and say, "Do this," and Wolfie, just a beginner then, would stare at his dad, and say, "I can't do that. You're Eddie Van Halen."

As I listen to the interview, I remember the way Ed used to sit Wolfie on his lap and play the piano, his fingers dancing across the keys much to the delight of his toddler son. The piano was in our library. Ed loved playing in there. One day he thanked me for creating a room with perfect acoustics. I was surprised. *I did? Well . . . cool.*

As time moves forward, the tears ebb into a more manageable and familiar flow. The holidays are hard, especially when I have the urge to call or text Ed and realize I can't even though his number is still in my phone along with years of texts. I work on recalibrating this change; Ed is gone but still so present. He is all over the Internet. With David. With Sammy. With Wolfie. His jaw-dropping solos. His underrated piano playing. That music will be around forever. Ed ain't going anyplace.

He shows up in my head, too. Our wedding. His cars. The craziness. The way we hurt each other. The birthdays. The phone calls. The tours. The way he turned to me and smiled while I was watching from the side of the stage thirty-five years ago because we were a couple but more recently because we were amazed by our kid. The man who blew away so many people with his musical virtuosity was blown away by his son. And I loved it. The debate between past and present is endless and unresolved.

· · · · · · · · ·

Love always wins.

That's why it hurts so badly.

Grief is one of those things you have to wade into and expect to cry your way to shallower waters.

Talking and remembering helps. Pictures are stepping-stones. Nighttime isn't as scary as those hours when you were accustomed to the phone ringing and hearing that familiar voice say hello or hey, what's happening.

I am doing exactly what Angie Johnsey advised nearly a year

earlier: acknowledge the voice in my head, address it, and put it where it belongs.

The sadness doesn't go away as much as I get better at dealing with it. I recognize it, speak to it, and use it. The grief seems to hit hardest when my tank is low, but instead of letting it knock me down, I use it to fill me up again. Someone should make a T-shirt that says, EMOTIONS ARE A TERRIBLE THING TO AVOID.

. . . . . . . . .

I find myself wanting to cook — not to eat but to create, connect, and share with others. One day I make my four-cheese crab mac 'n' cheese, a mouth-watering recipe that has two cups of cheddar cheese, a cup of Gruyère, a cup of fontina, some shredded Parmesan, and a pound of jumbo lump crabmeat topped by panko crumbs and scallions. A few weeks later, I have a yen for my kale Caesar salad with garlicky panko crunch. After finishing the dressing, with fresh garlic and anchovies, I declare it a punch to the tastebuds. All alone in the kitchen, I exclaim, "Yes!"

Later, I post a video of myself making this salad again on my Instagram. Faith Ford calls it a "yum explosion" in the comments section. It is, it is — and her reaction makes me feel lighter and brighter. This is more satisfying than the way I used to deal with my emotions. I am in the kitchen. The lights are on, there is no sneaking, no judgment, no labeling myself as bad. Where is Hoda? Savannah? Carson? I wish they were here to see me not crying for once but experiencing joy instead. And wanting seconds.

*More, please.*

Inspired, I go scrolling on my social media for more of what makes people happy. What are people's recipes for joy? This is some of what I find.

- My family
- A sunny day
- Laughing
- Hearing my child's voice (he's forty-seven years old and in the military, but he's still my baby)
- The doctor telling me that my husband made it through surgery
- Hearing "It's benign!"
- Music
- A glass of chilled white wine on the patio
- Making a stranger smile
- The smell of fresh bread
- Summer
- Offering someone a freshly baked chocolate chip cookie and seeing their reaction
- Family and friends
- Hearing Betty White tell a dirty joke
- My husband
- My wife
- My daughters
- Snuggling with my dogs
- Family dinners
- Sundays
- The quiet in church
- A walk on the beach
- My photo albums
- Cuddling in bed when it rains
- Puppies
- The smell of freshly cut grass
- Getting a hug when I need one, giving a hug when someone else needs one

- Working in my garden
- A good book on a lazy afternoon
- A nap — and at my age!
- Remembering the way my mom used to say, "Dinner-time!"
- Driving a new pet home from the shelter
- Calling my parents and being able to say, "Hi, Mom."
- Dancing
- My nonna turning ninety-nine
- Pizza
- Fishing with my dad (I'm a girl!)
- Holding hands
- Paying it forward
- My sobriety
- Paying someone's bill in a restaurant without telling them
- A hot fudge sundae — and it's been that way for seventy-four years
- Helping someone out of a jam
- A great song
- Listening to Maya Angelou read her poetry
- My kitty
- Good vibes
- Stephen King
- Room for my suitcase above my seat
- Going for a long run
- Nature
- A good joke
- An old tree
- Family get-togethers
- The smell of freshly cut flowers
- Tipping more than expected

- Knowing my husband is in remission
- Lending a hand
- Seeing people share and get along
- Legal weed
- Knees that bend without pain
- Work that I love
- Watching my children grow and find their joy
- Grandbabies
- Remembering my first kiss — and I married her!
- Seeing dolphins and whales, and knowing we aren't the only ones on this planet
- Volunteering at the food bank
- Spring
- Falling in love
- Seeing people love and care for each other
- Playing the piano
- Reese's peanut butter cups
- The Grand Canyon
- My twin
- My gray hair — I earned it!
- Remembering the way I partied at Van Halen in the eighties (oddly, I can't remember how I got home that night)
- Taking it one day at a time
- Being here
- Opening my eyes in the morning
- A goodnight kiss
- Saying I love you

So this is what I have learned the past year since going on the *Today* show and announcing that I want to experience joy. Joy is available to anyone who wants it without having to fix or change anything about yourself except your intention to make it a part of your life. It doesn't depend on losing ten pounds. It doesn't require luck. The pursuit of joy must be intentional and made a priority. There is no one path or recipe. In the end, there is just love. The search is like waking up groggy. You have to work through it. Feel your way, have your coffee, sit in the sun, and look around. Joy will not find you. But you can find it.

Somehow this has proved true during the strangest, saddest year of my adult life. I have discovered love in the midst of grief. I have found joy while crying a river of tears. Our lives are tapestries woven from various shades of joy and grief, happiness and pain, pleasure and disappointment, clarity and confusion, hope and fear, loneliness, longing, and love. You need all of it to understand any of it.

# A New Season

T HE THING I KNOW about gray skies is that they eventually clear. I am sure this is why the nightly local TV news is built around the seven-day weather report and why I check my Dark Sky weather app in the morning and again before I go to bed. Though it is possible to get a reasonably accurate sense of the weather simply by looking out the window, a seven- or ten-day forecast is similar to therapy.

It centers me. It reminds me and everyone else addicted to AccuWeather forecasts and Mega Doppler maps that things change. Every day is new and different.

We get through the cold and the storms. The sun will shine again.

*Patience.*

I have been telling myself this for a couple of weeks now. It is January, and I have made it through the holidays. It has not been easy. My eyes were closed much of the time. Once New Year's passed, I felt relief. This was true for most people: 2020 sucked. When I flipped my calendar, I thought about burning a bundle of sage.

I am supposed to be brainstorming ideas and recipes for the new season of *Valerie's Home Cooking*, our twelfth. It is scheduled to begin shooting in February. Despite creating a beautiful workplace where I have set out my mom's cookbooks and her recipe box for inspiration, I have been unable to concentrate. My brain is fogged in. Ideas are being told to circle until my head clears. It is always this way as we get close to production, but this time it's worse.

I worry that I have forgotten how to stand in front of cameras and cook. Rather than address that anxiety, I stew in it. I read novels. I make a lot of tea. I post about Wolfie's new music. I go on a knitting tear. I dye my hair blonde. Then I add a few streaks of pink. One day it rains, and I watch Henry and Luna sleep while researching the differences between two bottles of wine that have been sitting on my desk for a couple of months, one a Petite Sirah and the other a Syrah.

I don't know why I put myself through this torture, but I do. Not even Chrissy Teigen's Instagram can snap me out of this rut. The woman is a human energy drink; normally her posts provide the spark of inspiration I need to get started. But not this time, and I know the reasons. Losing Ed. Watching Wolfie grieve and not being able to fix it. The holidays. I slipped into the doldrums and can't get out. My weight is up, and I have a pain just below my neck and behind my right shoulder blade that feels like Spock's Vulcan nerve pinch.

One morning, as I sit in the library, I glance up and see Ed's beat-up Dr. Martens still on the shelf. Yes, still there. I can't believe myself sometimes. It's despite my best intentions, despite my best efforts, you know?

I look skyward and sigh. "Okay, kick my ass. I need it."

Later that afternoon, a friend comes over for a rare socially distanced visit. How long has it been since I sat across from someone who wasn't a family member? I set out a tray of snacks—some charcuterie, cheese, pickled okra, crackers, and pretzels—and open the bottle of Syrah. During our catch-up, she senses my sluggishness and asks when I last saw my therapist.

"Not for a while," I say. "Is it apparent?"

She takes a sip of wine and nods.

"What are you doing about your neck?" she asks.

"I need to find a chiropractor," I say.

"I'll give you the name of mine," she said. "She doesn't crack anything."

"What does she do?"

"She adjusts whatever needs adjusting."

"How?"

"Massage. And energy work."

"Energy work?"

"She's a little woo-woo."

"I need some woo-woo," I say.

. . . . . . . . .

An appointment with my therapist is first up. I haven't seen her since before Ed passed—a mistake, no doubt—and we have a productive session. She helps me peel back the layers until our roles seem reversed and I am explaining the problem to her. *I'm stuck, and I'm not doing the things to get myself unstuck.* Then I articulate the steps I need to take to get unstuck. *Don't isolate. Cut out snacks. Have one glass of wine instead of three. Get outside. Move my butt. And align with the things I love. Joy won't find me if I am locked in a dark room.*

A few days later, I am in the chiropractor's office. Since this is the first time I have seen her, I enter tentatively, wearing a mask, of course, and she takes my temperature and assures me that she is healthy and following protocols, too. Wearing the thick wooden clogs she put on my feet, I am soon lying facedown on her cushioned massage table and crying buckets of tears into my mask while she gently works on my legs and torso, muttering something to herself about my life force.

"Do most of your patients cry the first time they see you?" I ask.

She might have responded, but any memory of that is erased by what she tells me a few minutes later. While continuing to poke and press my back, legs, and neck, she mentions that my top rib is out of place and responsible for my neck and shoulder pain, which strikes me as weird but nowhere near as weird as when she says that we aren't alone.

"Huh?" I say, speaking directly into the hole in the face rest where my chin and mouth fit.

"I feel your mom in the room," she explains.

My first reaction is *What? My mom is here?* Then I feel a twinge of guilt because I haven't thought about my mom that much lately. I did have a dream about her recently, a lovely dream in fact, but I keep that to myself, saving it for my next session with my therapist.

"Oh?" I say. "My mom?"

"Yes. I might feel your dad, too," she says. "But he is nowhere near as strong as the female presence."

"What does she want?" I ask. "Is she saying anything?"

"She wants you to know it's all okay."

"Okay," I respond, but I am thinking — and refrain from asking — *Why don't you see Ed? Why isn't he here?*

After the session, I definitely feel better. The pain isn't entirely gone but it is less severe and I have more mobility in my neck. I make another appointment. Actually, I make one more for this week and two for the following week. On my drive home, I feel dizzy and light-headed even though she never came close to cracking my neck, which would release a vertiginous flood of toxins, as other chiropractors have done in the past.

Hours later, I am still thinking about that session. I enjoyed the woo-woo but am wondering what it means that my mom was there. What did she mean by *It's all okay*? Is she with me now? Is she always with me? I know that there is more to life than we are able to see. I know some people see more than others. When I look in the mirror, I see things in myself that are invisible to others. When they look at me, they see things I can't see. Just because something is not visible to everyone does not mean it isn't real.

Indeed, after I get into bed, I see Ed. My bedroom is dark, and I think, *Oh there you are*. I know the way that sounds. But this isn't the first time he has paid me a visit. A few days after he died, I was lying in bed in that woozy state where I was half awake and almost asleep, and I felt a presence in the room and I knew it was him. I cried, and said, "I love you. I miss you. I hope you know how much you were loved."

It would have been so much easier to tell myself that I was making this up, but I saw him clearly. I heard him, too. He looked at me, and said, "Oh," in the cute, empathetic manner that was his way of reacting to sensitive moments. Then I felt pressure in the middle of my forehead, as if he were pressing on it with his finger. He had very distinctive hands, gorgeous hands, in fact, and I was sure he was telling me through this gesture that he was all right and that I shouldn't be sad — not too sad, anyway.

*It's going to be okay.*

The further I have gotten from that October night, the more I have asked myself, *Did that really happen?*

One day I even issued a challenge. I was at the beach, and I said, "Okay, Ed, if I ever see a green cat, you have to come visit me and tell me that everything is good."

However, after my mom showed up earlier today and told me the same thing—*It's going to be okay*—I have decided to quit asking. Things must be okay.

. . . . . . . . .

And they are. By the following week, the heaviness and anxiety that had rendered me immobile gradually lifts so I am able to get back on track, starting with the simplest of remedies—I move. Each morning after my coffee, I take a brisk walk through the neighborhood with Luna. I breathe in the crisp air and enjoy the blank slate of the day ahead. Birds chirp. Dew glistens on the leaves. The sun warms as it breaks through the clouds. The air is full of optimism and possibilities. It's like a happy drug. Why don't I do this more often?

I feel my heart pumping. My knees ache and my neck and back are reluctant participants, but they hurt a little less each day. I resist the urge to get on the scale. What's it going to tell me that I can't feel?

At home, I reward myself with a refreshing smoothie. I blend bananas, almond butter, almond milk, some rolled oats, honey, and the half a cup of coffee that more than anything else keeps the pep in my energy level. I pour it into a beautiful glass and top it off with a couple of sprigs of mint from my garden. Why not treat myself to a nice presentation? More to the point, why not treat myself nicely?

It makes a difference. Not only am I eager to work when I sit down at my desk, I am also filled with gratitude. I was so mired in woe-is-me before that I overlooked this key ingredient. *Valerie's Home Cooking* is about home cooking at a time when everyone in the world is at home cooking and craving the comfort of delicious, simple meals. I can almost hear Norman Lear telling the fifteen-year-old me to "go get 'em, kid." Except it's my mom, my Non-nie, and my great-grandmother who are giving me the thumbs-up.

In so many ways, it really is a new season—for the show, for me, for everyone. Life is one big table where we are supposed to feed and nourish one another. "Pull up a chair," the great food writer Ruth Reichl once wrote. "Take a taste."

Ideas come to me. A new Bolognese for a simpler lasagna. Ham, apple, and cheddar sliders. A jar of marinara sauce on my kitchen counter inspires a fairly traditional baked ziti with a mix of sliced vegetables that I throw together in my slow cooker. I fish into my mom's recipe box and pull out the well-worn card for her onion rings. I make them—and forget them in the oven, where they cook for way too long. Wolfie dubs them *overdonion rings.*

"But they're delicious," he says.

My first production meeting with Mary Beth Bray, now an executive producer, and culinary producer Sophie Clark is on Zoom and I am eager to share my ideas. Choosing the menus for each episode is my favorite part of the show. But before we dive into the recipes and organize them into individual episodes, we have so much catching up to do. We haven't been together since March 2020 when we cut the previous season short by three episodes and bid one another a hasty goodbye because of the shutdown.

"How's everyone doing?" I say. "It's so good to see your faces. I've missed you."

During the break, Mary Beth moved with her family to LA from New York. She shares some details about their cross-country drive, most of them involving little places they stopped to eat and her delicious discoveries along the way. Sophie and I take notes.

The episodes come together quickly. Recipes range from lemony *cacio e pepe* and homemade pretzel buns with butter and ham to salmon sliders and buffalo chicken burgers to a spring roll salad with peanut butter dressing and a quinoa, sweet potato, and black bean bowl with cilantro yogurt dressing. The sweets include orange vanilla bean angel food cake, no-bake chocolate peanut butter bars, no-churn lemon ice cream, and almond butter, oat, and cranberry cookies.

Even though the shows are supposed to be timeless, I want to address Covid and talk directly to viewers about being in the kitchen more this past year, and everyone agrees that this makes sense. So we schedule my friend, food writer Jo Stougaard, as my guest on the first episode. Her nephew is a firefighter and his wife is a nurse. I will put together a picnic basket for Jo to take to them. Smoked-turkey sandwiches with Calabrian chili aioli, homemade salt and vinegar potato chips, and s'mores that don't need a campfire.

The show is shot at a house with a remodeled kitchen. I am buzzing with happiness and excitement from being back on the set. Almost everyone involved with the production has been part of the show since day one. Before starting, we gather in the backyard. All of us are masked; everyone has been tested. I thank everyone for their contributions. The show would be impossible to do otherwise. Mary Beth echoes those sentiments, expressing gratitude for the good health we have all enjoyed.

"It's a new season," she says. "Let's have fun."

. . . . . . . . .

By April, all the episodes have been shot and are being edited. The show has also been picked up for a thirteenth season. I know I won't be as tortured this next time. In addition to keeping up my morning walks and concocting new flavors for my smoothies, I have added an afternoon workout — twenty to forty-five minutes on my Peloton bike. In a break from the past, the workout didn't start as a punishment for being overweight, though I am not happy with my weight right now. The difference is that I don't hate myself. I have been feeling good and I wanted to feel better. My body actually craved the exercise, and I was happy to oblige.

It has been six months since Ed passed, and every day I am learning that grief doesn't go away as much as it evolves into something manageable. I will still burst into tears when Wolfie has a question or a problem and my first thought is *Well, let's call your dad*—and, of course, we can't. Other times, I am awash in happy memories that I wear like a piece of jewelry, knowing that they make me shine. Then there are those days when I forget and go about my business until I stumble over a reminder.

That's what happened last night.

I got into bed and was scrolling through TikTok, as I sometimes do. Just before I put my phone on my nightstand, something on the screen caught my attention. It was a little green dump truck. Inside the truck were three little kitties. I remembered the challenge I had issued to Ed a few months ago. *If I see a green cat, you have to visit me again.* Did kittens in a green toy dump truck count? I was too sleepy to laugh, but I thought, *How silly*, then turned off my phone, pulled up the covers, settled into my pillows, and shut my eyes.

I don't know how much time elapsed, whether it was seconds, minutes, or hours, but I was drifting in that half-asleep, half-awake place when I sensed a presence in the room. I opened my eyes and there, through the darkness, was Ed. Looking at me. With that Cheshire cat grin of his. *Like you asked for it. Here I am.*

"What's going on?" I asked. "Are you really here?"

Ed didn't speak. But all of a sudden, I felt my body pulled down from my pillows into the bed, then, whoosh, I felt like I was being carried up through the roof into the night sky where I saw the stars twinkling and sparkling into infinity, a celestial light show that was beautiful, bright, thrilling, and endless. It was as if I were being asked, *You wanted to experience joy. What do you think of this?*

Then I found myself back in bed, still sleepy or perhaps fully asleep, I don't know for sure. But I felt extremely calm, warm, comfortable, and curious.

"Is this you? Are you here?" I asked again.

No answer.

"Okay, if you're here, play it for me. Only you will know what I'm talking about. So play it for me."

Up in the corner of the room, by the ceiling, there was a flash of light. I turned my head and saw a tiny screen. It was followed by the sound of a guitar. By this time, I was half expecting to see Patrick Swayze hovering over Demi Moore at a potter's wheel. But no, I heard only the sound of a guitar that was unmistakably Ed playing a hybrid of the intro to "Women in Love . . ." and Wolfie's song "Think It Over." It was a completely unique mash-up as only Ed could do, a little something that I loved combined with something he loved, and I knew that he was doing it especially for me.

When he finished, the tiny light disappeared and he picked me up again and floated me around the room one more time before setting me down in the bed. At this point, I didn't need any more proof. Some things you can't explain and don't want or need them to be explained, and this was one of those things. I leaned forward to give him a kiss and felt not only the stubble on his face but also the pressure of someone hugging me.

"I love you," I said, as I slipped into a deep sleep.

I never heard his voice, but I woke up with a clear sense that not only were things okay, good things were also going to come.

· · · · · · · · ·

Listen, I hear how crazy this sounds. I do. And maybe it was all just a dream. But it felt real to me—and whatever gets us through these hard times. You know?

Now here's the kicker. After spending the rest of today thinking about what happened and wondering how I could know all those details if it didn't really happen, and also feeling really good about everything, I have sent word to Ed. *Last night was amazing and special, and I definitely want to see you again but not tonight. I am sixty —almost sixty-one—and I am worn-out. I can't go flying around the stars every night.*

# The Little Girl Needs a Hug

### APRIL 2021

S TOP EVERYTHING. I HAVE got breaking news. I think there is a very good chance that I am an innately happy, joyful person who just needed sixty-one years to recognize it.

Gawd, I am thinking what a doofus I have been. Time is too precious to have wasted so much of it.

Let me try to explain what *finally* happened.

## 1. Don't laugh, but it starts with cat videos

Almost every morning before I get out of bed, I watch cat videos on TikTok. I am not alone in this habit. It is a genuine phenomenon accounting for billions of views. Over the years, researchers have observed actual therapeutic benefits from watching cat videos, like helping people relax and de-stress. An entry on Wikipedia even claims that "feelings of guilt when postponing tasks can be reduced by watching cat videos."

In other words, watching cat videos makes procrastinators like me feel okay about procrastinating. Left unsaid is the reason we are procrastinating. It is because we are watching cat videos. I suppose that as long as the house isn't burning down our love for cats takes precedence over practically everything.

Because of this habit of watching cat videos, I meander into other areas of TikTok one day. There, amid the dancers and singers, the cute babies, and Zach King's mind-blowing illusions, I come upon the deja vu challenge, where TikTok users post videos of themselves lip-synching to Olivia Rodrigo's song "Deja Vu" while using the app's inverted filter to toggle back and forth between their mirror image and an inverted image of themselves. This inverted image apparently shows the way other people really see you.

It is mostly girls and young women doing this, and many of them are supposedly having a hard time seeing the inverted image of themselves. In theory, that is because this is something we never see and remain oblivious to—our true selves. Typically, we only see ourselves in photographs or a mirror. A mirror shows us a reverse image of ourselves and only confirms whatever we are accustomed to telling ourselves that we see or want to see.

The inverted filter, however, shows a different view, the one that other people see when they look at us. It eliminates our personal biases toward ourselves and supposedly portrays who we really are.

I am intrigued.

I obviously have issues.

I have been trying to deal with exactly this issue since I went on the *Today* show almost a year and a half ago, and basically said, "Enough already. How do I get on with my life and experience joy in the body I have right now?" That doesn't mean I am content with the way I look. Yes, I have to lose a few pounds. I might have to cut down on some food, give up an extra glass of wine, and get on my bike another day or two each week. I want to be healthy. But I don't want to torture myself anymore. At this age, I can't be as flawed as I constantly tell myself I am, at least not to the point where it prevents me from enjoying everything else.

And, of course, everyone tells me that I am right, that I am smart, funny, and beautiful. Or they simply say, "You are crazy."

And Angie Johnsey has given me tools to deal with the voice in my head that always says, "you need to lose ten pounds and then . . ."

And I feel like I am making progress.

But for some reason, I still pay more attention to those who troll me on the Internet instead of the people who compliment the photos and videos I post. Why do I give credence to the haters? Why don't I believe the nice people?

I know why. Old habits die hard. The negative comments are easier to believe. They confirm the negative things I have always told myself. How could I possibly believe people who say I am beautiful when I don't see that myself?

Which is what makes me super curious about and maybe a tad scared of this inverted filter. How do other people see me? How will I react to seeing myself that way?

I have no idea what I am going to see when I pull out my phone, log into TikTok, and shoot a video of myself using the inverted filter. Am I going to cry the way some people have when they see themselves? ("OMG, in tears! Is that how ppl really see me?") Am I going to see confirmation of all the things the haters have seen and said over the years? I don't have any makeup on and my hair is pulled back. I look the way I do when I finish working out and am flushed, sweaty, plain, and, in my opinion, at my ugliest.

The video is less than one minute long. When I watch it for the first time, I gasp. "Oh my God, I'm my mom!" I shriek.

I see a flash of her and shudder from the shock of recognition.

Then I watch it again. And then again. After the third time, I push pause and stare at the screen, where I see myself, not my mom, and for the first time in as long as I can remember, I think, *I'm not ugly*.

It is a revelation. *I'm not ugly*.

I tear up. *I'm not ugly*.

I know it sounds odd that a short video on a gimmicky app can have this effect, but it does. It frees something inside me. I feel like I have stepped outside and seen sunlight for the first time in a while. And in that brief flash, I see myself. For the first time in my life, I glimpse what others see when they look at me and . . .

## 2. I am going to skip that part for a moment

Life gets busy to the point where I can feel normal creeping into the picture. I get my second Covid vaccination the week before my birthday. No reaction, but I take it easy. Over the weekend, Wolfie sits on the floor signing several thousand copies of his album, which will be released in June, and Patrick and I put them back in the large brown boxes they came in. It's like we are running a mom-and-pop operation. I have to prep for a cooking demo for the USO. Then I meet with my producer and culinary producer to begin planning season thirteen of *Valerie's Home Cooking*.

For my birthday, Wolfie comes over with a box of cupcakes from SusieCakes. The box also contains two slices of their lemon cake, my favorite. I want to remember this picture of me celebrating sixty-one. My smile is more genuine than the one millions of people saw more than a decade ago when I was in a bikini. BIKINI BOD AT 48! screamed the headline on the cover of *People* magazine, as if the editors couldn't believe I had lost more than forty pounds and gotten in the best shape of my life.

But looks are deceiving. I had to practically starve myself the week before the photo shoot in order to feel comfortable getting into a bikini, and I obviously didn't keep the weight off. I mean, look at me. I started to gain it back as soon as that shoot wrapped. Would I ever go to that extreme again? No way. I have figured out something else, something different and healthier for me in the long run. I feel guilty about the message I put out to people back then. I was part of the problem of diet culture and making women feel less than good about themselves unless they hit a certain number on the scale.

Hey, I wasn't immune to it myself. Even as I dieted and exercised like an Olympic athlete, I was made to feel bad if I had a little pooch on the side or was a little heavier than my targeted weight that week. The whole experience opened my eyes to realities I had not thought about before. Like the way so many people in the health-diet-beauty industries market to our insecurities. Like the way the fashion industry's inconsistencies in sizing make us feel terrible. It's like they keep moving the goalposts. In her day, Marilyn Monroe was a size sixteen. She would be a six today. What's the deal? She was five-six and one hundred twenty pounds. I can't think of a more beautiful woman. She was all curvy and all natural.

As long as I am ranting, why do we use the term "plus-size model"? If we do that, why don't we also have a term like "super tiny and skinny model"? Why do we have to label and judge? Full-size, mid-size, husky — these words have been warped and weaponized. Sizes should be universal, guilt free, and created and maintained to do one thing, help people pull clothing from the shelf that fits their body and makes them feel good about it.

I am obviously a bit frothy over this. I am not even sure how to articulate the way I feel about all this and my role in it other than to say I'm sorry and explain that I was under the same influence as everyone else. I put out a message that I was only going to feel good if I lost x number of pounds and got into a bikini. I believed it, too. Then the big reveal not only put pressure on me, it also made others look critically at their own body and think of themselves as not bikini ready when the truth is that there is no such thing as bikini ready or a beach body. I repeat: *There is no such thing*. And I am sorry if I led people to believe that there was.

I have a friend whose daughter is a therapist who works with women and girls who have body and food issues, and she gives them a simple and clear message when it comes to being beach and swimsuit ready: "Get dressed—and if you're okay with the level of camel toe, there's no nip slip, and you don't have food in your teeth, you're good to go."

I have a simpler message. Do what makes you feel good about yourself. Don't strive to be anything other than who you are naturally. You can work out. You can lose weight. God knows I try to do both, and I have been succeeding more often than not lately. But don't confuse that with dieting. I take care of myself in a way that suits my lifestyle and my mental health, which means addressing not the weight but the pain and sadness I see in the mirror, and knowing that if I do that I will arrive naturally at the best weight for me.

**3. Two weeks after my second vaccination, I meet my girlfriends for a belated birthday dinner at Casa Vega, our favorite neighborhood Mexican restaurant**

It is the first time any of us have been together in more than a year. We sit outside and eat, talk, and toast one another with margaritas for several hours. Being together in person, laughing and trading smiles, is like having oxygen pumped into my lungs. At the end of the night, we stand in the parking lot and hug one another, not really wanting to let the night go or let go of one another.

*I missed you.*

*I love you.*

*I can't believe it's been more than a year.*

*I love you.*

*I love you.*

All of us are in our sixties. We sound like a bunch of fifth grade girls who have gone out to dinner without our parents and have had the best time ever.

At home, I am still glowing as I get ready for bed. I wash my face and get into my pj's. I think I might read for a bit, but when I reach for the book on my nightstand, my hand falls on my phone instead. I know you aren't supposed to keep your phone that close to your bed. I do anyway. It's the teenager in me. Something might happen; I will need to know instantly. In the morning, I will need to take a picture of the cats stretched out across the bed. About the only thing I won't use it for is to make or answer a call. Hey, we all have our quirks.

My intention is to watch a few cat videos on TikTok. But I click on my own TikTok video. I want to see if I have the same reaction to it as two weeks ago. This time it is even better. I don't just see someone who isn't ugly. I see someone I like. I see eyes that are full of kindness. I see my vulnerability. I see someone who tried to be a good daughter and sister. I see someone who did a good job being a mom. I see someone who works hard. I see someone who has a good sense of humor. I see someone who knows how to laugh and laugh loudly. I see someone who is a good sport. I see someone who cares. I see someone who has not always been her best but who has tried and continues to try. I see someone who wants to be a grandma. I also see a girl who needs to lose a few pounds. At the same time, I see someone who is coming alive—finally.

I think I see what other people might see, the strangers who always say they can relate to me; I think I see the kind of person who doesn't have to pretend to have it all together, who is a real human being, not perfect and not even trying to be perfect, just trying to be good. I see the kindness in my eyes.

I also see someone who is trying to be her authentic self. No makeup. Hair pulled back. Clear eyes. And she's smiling. She's a little girl—the little girl who has always tried to entertain and make people feel good. Only the voices are no longer telling her to do that. She's just being herself. I see that she wants a hug. She needs a hug.

I give her a hug, and I know that as long as I keep hugging her she will get stronger. She just needs love. It always comes back to love.

I delete the video, turn off the light, and get myself comfy in bed. I am going to have a good sleep.

## 4. I guest on *The Secret Life of Cookies* podcast

During the podcast, the host, Marissa Rothkopf, a wonderful writer about food, compliments me for being a person who exudes happiness, and she asks me how and why that is, if I have always been that way. Instead of my usual glib retort, "Well, you just choose happy," I offer a bit of what this past year has been like and the way I have worked to clear up the pigpen of messages that has resided in my head for much of my life (picture Charlie Brown's pal), and in doing so, in hearing myself babble on, I come to realize that (a) I like this voice, I really like this voice that is in my head and coming out of my mouth, and (b) joy and happiness might truly be my innate default setting.

Other people have always seen it, and now, with the work I have been doing since I met Angie plus all the other crap that has forced me to take a long, hard, and honest look at the way I see myself today, at this age, in this body, I am ready to embrace myself as joyful and happy. I am ready to own it and pursue it while knowing that some days will be harder than others but that it's always within reach. It is always inside me. It's always been there. It is my default setting. But now I can hear it.

A little later, I sit down with a glass of wonderful chardonnay, and I say to myself, *Huh, you know what? I am happy.*

I know that sounds friggin' weird.

It feels weird, too.

It also feels great.

# The House I Want to Die In

## MAY 2021

WELCOME TO MY BEACH house. The four-bedroom Cape Cod–style home sits atop a cliff, though you wouldn't know that from the street. But pass through the door between the garage and the guest house and you come face-to-face with a view that stops people in their tracks. It happens every time no matter how often people have been here, including to me —and I bought the house in 1984 back when I was twenty-four years old, had few expenses, and could afford it after a decade on a top-rated TV series.

A long, steep staircase leads down to the sand. Wherever you stand, it's a genuine wow, especially when the dolphins and whales swim within view, which is fairly often. It's as if they know us and come by to say, *Hey, what's up?* Even with your eyes closed, you can hear the waves, and when the swells get big and break hard, the ground shakes, and once again you can't help but stop and exclaim, "Wow!"

I drove here yesterday and met up with Wolfie, Andraia, Patrick, and Stacy, all of whom have been staying here for a while. I have no idea how long they have been here and they have lost track, too, which happens at the beach. Patrick says it's impossible to be productive here, and he's right. Your head goes into vacation mode, and your body operates in slow motion. Everything takes thirty minutes longer. Except for cocktail hour. Somehow that gets earlier and earlier.

But I have an agenda that includes more than chilling. Despite the magnificent setting, the house is in desperate need of work. Pipes leak, some rooms have water damage and mold, and there are major structural issues; that's on top of the corrosion from exposure to sun, wind, fog, and salt water plus the problems of age. In its present state, the house reminds me of a senior citizen who, after suffering through one of those terrible, convulsive coughing fits, realizes that she made a tactical error by going decades without seeing her doctor.

The neglect is my fault. Like everything else in my life, I let the problems pile up until they took over. That's about to change finally. Years of work and conversations with my architect have turned into an actual plan. At the end of the summer, the existing house will be torn down and a brand-new house will be erected. It has taken three years for me to come to terms with the design. Pictures of my architect's renderings are on my phone. That's the reason I have driven to the beach. I am ready to show them to Wolfie and my brother.

Why it has taken me so long is typical of me. Actually, given the pace at which I normally move, this timeline is downright brisk. How it happened is also a perfect reflection of what I have been going through and where I hope to be. About five years ago, I was looking for something in the kitchen. I opened several drawers and was overwhelmed by clutter. The same thing happened when I looked through the cabinets. There was too much stuff— too much that I didn't need or want crammed into every available space. Ultimately, I gave up my search and decided I had to redo the kitchen—and maybe a few other rooms.

I met with my architect, the same person who redid my house in the hills, so he knew me well and knew what he was getting into. I was honest and transparent as I showed him around, explaining that the house had a lot of problems I had let pile up over the years. I might as well have been talking to my therapist as I discussed what worked, what didn't work, what I liked about the house, what I didn't like, and the things I wanted to change. It was my life.

"I've let some things go," I said.

"Everyone does." He smiled.

"I was pregnant with Wolfie the last time I redid anything here."

"How old is he now?"

"Almost thirty."

"Wow, then it's time." He smiled again.

"I love this house," I said. "I don't even know how much needs to be changed."

"How much do you want to change?" he asked.

"We can tear down some walls. But I don't want to change the footprint."

"Okay. The footprint stays. It works for you."

"Yes."

"What doesn't work for you?"

· · · · · · · · ·

Thank goodness he already knew how painful change of any type was for me. But this house was in a category of its own. I was deeply sentimental about it and intent on holding on to its past. So much had happened in it. When I first saw it, I fell in love instantly. The house was empty. It had been rebuilt after a recent wildfire had roared down the hills, jumped Pacific Coast Highway, and burned it and the neighboring homes.

But I sensed that it was in shock. I promised to take care of it and fill it with full and happy lives. At first, my parents lived there full-time. My brothers and their wives came and went. Ed and I were there on weekends and holidays. In 1985, I suffered a miscarriage in the upstairs bedroom. A few years later, my dad and Ed got into their infamous fistfight there. Dad and Patrick painted and repainted the exterior numerous times. Even after I changed the original blue color to yellow, I referred to it as the "blue house." We threw great Super Bowl parties there, played volleyball, and romped on the beach.

I threw Ed a surprise thirtieth birthday party in this house, but we arrived four hours late because I couldn't get him out of the studio. "Why do I have to go all the way out to the beach to celebrate my birthday?" he kept asking. I wanted to clobber him. I can still hear myself sneaking a phone call to the house. "We still haven't left yet."

"But you said that two hours ago."

"Tell that to the birthday boy."

MTV shot here before Van Halen went to Cabo. Sammy Hagar bought a house two doors up. It was a great place to hang out and decompress, which Ed did so well here. Patrick would marvel at the way Ed could lie on the sofa watching TV with a guitar on his lap while playing "the most insane stuff without even seeming to think about what he was doing. He wasn't even paying attention," my brother would say. "And yet you could see him staring off into the distance pulling these ideas in from some other planet."

After Wolfie started kindergarten and I became friendly with some of the other moms, this became the perfect spot for us to meet on a Friday afternoon and sit on the cliff with a glass of wine and watch the sun set while our kids played in the yard. When Ed and I divorced, he kept the Coldwater Canyon house with the studio and I got the beach house, but I still let him use it whenever he wanted. One time I went out the day after he had been there and found that he had forgotten to turn off the burner on the stove. He felt terrible. He could have burned down the house—along with the entire neighborhood.

I married Tom on the patio on January 1, 2011. Ed was there that night, along with my parents, my brothers, and my dearest friends. Everyone in my life has been there and helped create memories, and when I look around, I can still see and hear them. I can go there, sit on the bluff, and feel my parents. I can talk with Ed. I can see Wolfie running around with his friends. Everyone is still there. And that's what has scared me most about this remodeling project. I can be alone there and I am still with the people I love.

I am fine with adding new people and new memories, but I don't want to lose anything from the past. I can't let go.

. . . . . . . . .

"That's always the problem," my architect said. "What do you keep? What do you change? What do you throw out altogether?"

We were seated at the dining-room table, and he was about to show me his new plans for the first time. He pushed his iPad toward me, explaining that he had created three-dimensional animations of the new house that would let me visualize the street view outside and the different rooms inside, including the view of the ocean from various balconies. Nervous, I took a deep breath and began to scroll. Moments later, I started to cry. Neither of us had expected that reaction. I think I went into shock.

"It's not my house," I said. "It's not the blue house."

Not even close. From the front, it looked like the exterior of a covered bridge in the Vermont countryside. The back was wide open, modern, and barnlike, an homage to family and the outdoors done in wood and glass. Inside, everything was about light and space and seeing the ocean, with numerous spots for gathering, including a ground-level patio that seemed to flow out of the kitchen and reminded me of alfresco dining in Italy via Malibu.

When I finished going through the pictures, my tears were replaced by a look of awe and I was speechless. It was one of those rare moments when the future reveals itself, and though I was not ready to commit to anything definitive, I liked what I saw. Not only was I impressed, I was also excited—and scared. My architect had studied me, listened to me, and returned with his interpretation of my journey from the time I had purchased the house to the present. He gave me a picture that showed change, growth, and possibilities.

Actually, what he did was show me my potential.

"I love it, I think," I said. "It scares me. In a good way. But I want to sit with it for a while."

. . . . . . . . .

A while turned out to be three years. Now I am ready to show Wolfie and my brother. It is Sunday afternoon, and the sun is out and turning the ocean into a display of sparkling diamonds. Wolfie is finishing an interview with a radio station, and Patrick and Stacy are getting ready to return to their home in Arizona. Barefoot in the kitchen, I set out a late lunch of grilled jalapeño peppers stuffed with ground turkey and cheese. Someone asks for hot sauce. Another wants water. I laugh. I am cook, waitress, mom, sister, and just plain Valerie—exactly as I like it, especially out here at the beach house.

Then it's time. I gather everyone around the table, remind them of the road that led to the pictures they are about to see, then I hand them my phone. At first, Wolfie and Patrick are quiet. They scroll through the animations without saying a word. Then they can't stop themselves from shouting one superlative after another. *Oh my God. Amazing. I can't believe it. Incredible.*

Wolfie envelops me in his arms and squeezes.

"It's so cool, Mom," he says.

"I know," I say. "It's . . . it's big."

It's not the only big change. There's the situation with Tom. We have separated. Fissures in the relationship surfaced years ago, and like what happened to nearly everyone I know, the lockdown led to a serious reassessment of priorities. What do I want versus what do I need? What is helping me move forward in my life? What is holding me back? I had started asking those questions before Covid and I am still asking them. In my search to experience more joy, I have to identify and move past ideas and behavior that no longer serve me, and my eleven-year marriage to Tom is one of those things.

The decision has been a slow, painful one. But we have drifted from the interests that made us a couple and found that those differences can't be fixed. He is a good man who is going through many of the same issues that I have faced: What can he do to add meaning and purpose to his life? Where can he find joy? What is he passionate about? What has he learned? And what does he do differently going forward?

The paths we thought we were on changed. It doesn't make us bad people. It means we are human. I want only the best for him. As for me, I know separating could mean that I spend the rest of my life on my own, and if that's the case, I am ready to try and will approach it without fear or regret. As many women will explain, being single doesn't mean being available. It doesn't mean unavailable, either. It can have a multitude of meanings, including independent, confident, content, adventurous, searching, questioning, working on things.

All of that is true, and I am ready to see what happens next.

I don't want to waste time anymore. This past year has shown me and everyone else how precious time really is. I stopped looking for a magic number. I turned sixty. My second marriage is ending. My first husband and soulmate died. I dealt with grief—my own and my son's. I went back to work. I got vaccinated. And I asked, *What have I learned from all of this? How have I changed? What am I going to try to do differently going forward?*

So many of us are feeling the same way and trying to figure out how we come out of this better and wiser. I think we got a good look at some serious problems that have been ignored for far too long and we know that it's time to fix them—and fix ourselves. I think we know that we are supposed to be better and kinder to one another.

· · · · · · · · ·

Later that afternoon, as we sit around talking and listening to the waves, Wolfie adds another special memory to the beach house when he tells me that he started writing his album here at the beach. I had no idea. When he got off the 2012 Van Halen tour, he moved out of his apartment and into the guest house here.

"I didn't want to live with either you or Dad," he says.

Moored out here in the middle of nowhere, he taught himself Logic Pro and wrote the song "Mammoth."

He asks if I want to hear the demo.

"Uh, yes," I say affirmatively. "Duh, I want to hear it."

Wolfie tries streaming it on the living-room speakers, but it won't play. He can't get it to play on the smaller kitchen speakers, either. His frustration comes out in a childish growl: "The Internet here is messed up." Eventually, he plays it on his phone and the original is not much different than the final version — a beautiful, powerful, and even upbeat song about dealing with depression.

"I love those lyrics," I say. *It's not okay to get up and walk away . . . anything is possible.*

"Thanks, Ma," he says.

"That's my boy," I say.

A second or two passes before I correct myself. I look out the window at the clouds crisscrossing the sky, and say silently, *Hey, I meant that's our boy.*

Then I get up and announce that I am going for a walk before dinner. I head toward the staircase leading to the beach. It is one hundred and four steps down to the sand, then one hundred and four steps back up. But you know what? It's time to quit counting the number of steps and just enjoy the friggin' walk.

You know what I mean?

*Pay attention to what really matters.*
*Don't change. Grow.*
*Be kind to yourself. Be kind to others.*
*Learn to forgive.*
*Be a helper, not a hater.*
*Be open to whatever happens next.*
*And look for love.*
*In the end, it's only and all about love.*

# Learning to Love the Way I Am Today

## *My To-Do List*

MAY 2021

1. Tidy your mind — stop thinking negative thoughts about yourself and others
2. Drink water
3. Exercise
4. Eat more vegetables and fruits than anything else
5. Serve others before (or at least as often as) you serve yourself
6. Practice kindness daily
7. Avoid trolls
8. Try new things and give yourself permission to fail
9. Work with intention
10. Grow
11. Help

12. Share
13. Laugh loudly and often
14. Live with gratitude
15. Love

# Pizza, Please

What more can I say? Live life. Play your music loud. And enjoy your pizza. Please.

## For the pizza

3½ cups bread flour, spooned and leveled

1½ teaspoons kosher salt

1½ teaspoons instant yeast

½ cup extra virgin olive oil, divided

1½ cups water, lukewarm

1 teaspoon honey

4 to 5 ounces sliced pepperoni

12 deli slices Monterey Jack cheese or provolone (about ½ pound)

8 ounces shredded mozzarella

Dried oregano, for garnish

Red pepper flakes, for garnish

Freshly grated Parmesan, for garnish

## For the sauce

1 14-ounce can crushed tomatoes

2 tablespoons extra virgin olive oil

1 clove garlic, grated

¾ teaspoon kosher salt

¼ teaspoon granulated sugar

*(recipe continued on next page)*

Add the flour, salt, and yeast to the bowl of a stand mixer and whisk to combine.

Add the water, 3 tablespoons of the olive oil, and the honey to a 2-cup measuring cup. Whisk to combine.

Add the water mixture to the mixer and use a rubber spatula to start to incorporate the ingredients.

Attach the bowl to the stand mixer, fit with the dough hook, and mix on low speed until the mixture forms into a ball and no loose flour is left at the base of the bowl, 3 to 4 minutes. Turn the mixer up to medium speed and knead for 2 to 3 minutes.

Pour the remaining olive oil into a 13-by-18 rimmed baking sheet.

Turn the dough out onto the baking sheet. Turn it once to coat all the sides of the dough in the olive oil.

Cover the pan with an inverted baking sheet and leave in a warm place to rise for 2 hours, until doubled in size.

After 2 hours, preheat the oven to 500 degrees F.

Remove the top baking sheet and, using the tips of your fingers, delicately stretch the dough until it almost reaches the edges of the pan. Cover again with the rimmed baking sheet and let the dough rest while you make the sauce.

Add the crushed tomatoes, the olive oil, grated garlic, salt, and sugar to a mixing bowl. Whisk to combine and set aside.

Uncover the dough and delicately stretch the dough to reach all the edges of the pan. If the dough springs back too much, let the dough sit for another 5 to 10 minutes before trying to stretch it again.

Once the dough is stretched to fit the pan, top it with the sauce. Cover the sauce completely with the pepperoni, then top the pepperoni with the sliced cheese and shredded mozzarella.

Transfer the pizza to the oven and bake for 15 to 20 minutes, until the cheese is lightly browned in spots and the crust is golden.

Remove the pizza from the oven and use a large spatula to transfer it to a cutting board. Top with dried oregano, red pepper flakes, and Parmesan. Cut into 16 squares and serve immediately.

**Prep time:** 2.5 hours (includes rising time)

**Cook time:** 15 to 20 minutes

**Serves** 6 people

# Acknowledgments

This book began as a way to address one issue and turned into something that I think and hope reflects numerous experiences that are familiar to many of us. It was hard to relive and share many of these memories. I have gone back and forth about whether I am revealing too much and being too open, and I have asked myself if that helps anyone. I ended up telling myself that while these are the details of my life everyone goes through similar things. I think sharing makes us feel less alone during the hardest of times and reminds us that the joy and happiness that make for best of times are the little things that we have to make a priority.

I think it helps to open up a book and find tips and advice and hear someone else say, "I don't have it all together but I'm doing my best and you can, too." And I really find it beneficial to know that people are on the sidelines rooting for me. And that is the way I think of you. I have been so privileged over my long career, now spanning almost fifty years; and the biggest gift has been you— and all the nice people who have grown up with me and feel like they know me. I want to say thank you for watching and reading and sending messages, and I want to let you know that I appreciate it and send the love and support right back to you. We are in this together and that is ultimately why I went ahead with this book. It's for all of us.

One idea that didn't change was my desire to write a book composed of numerous stories that could be opened and read at any point and that has familiar threads stitched throughout that will eventually get you, the reader, through it the same way I got through it. It was difficult to live and equally difficult to write, but in the end, I feel like I was able to say a few things that are always worth saying: People are beautiful from the inside out. Nobody is perfect. Kindness and forgiveness clear the skies, feed our souls, and help us sleep soundly. Life is precious. Don't waste it.

All of us know that living life is a group effort and writing a book like this is no different. I have so many people to thank, starting with my friend and frequent collaborator Todd, who sat with me for months during Covid, in our own little pod, and helped with this book. I appreciate how much we can get done when all we are doing is sitting in front of our laptops and talking to each other.

I want to thank my editor, Karen Murgolo, and publishers Deb Brody and Liate Stehlik, Jacqueline Quirk, Jennifer Freilach, Sara Alexander, Andrea DeWerd, and everyone at Houghton Mifflin Harcourt (now HarperCollins) for believing I had something to say and helping to get this labor of love to the finish line. Similarly, I want to thank my literary agents Dan Strone and Tess Weitzner of Trident Media Group, for helping yet again find my latest book — and me — the right home. A similarly big thank you to my longtime publicist, Jill Fritzo. And Zachary Bradshaw, who so kindly keeps my life in order. Marc Schwartz and Jack Grossbart are two special men who have been in my life professionally and personally for decades. They want the best for me, they have done their best for me, and they always have my best interests in mind. I may not say it enough but thank you.

I also need to acknowledge and thank everyone at the *Today* show, the producers behind the scenes and my friends in front of the camera. All of you started this journey that I didn't even realize I needed to be on. Angie Johnsey and Melissa Brohner-Schneider, you showed me the path and how to stay on it.

As all of us know, the kitchen is where the good stuff happens and gets discussed, and that is so true on *Valerie's Home Cooking*. I am immensely grateful to Mary Beth, Sophie, Lindsey, Susan, Pete, and the whole VHC crew—too numerous to name individually but all very much in my heart. Thank you. On the personal side, I want to express my adoration of the Vitale family. Robin, girl, you keep me sane. Tom, the time that I spent with you, that we spent together, helped me on the journey to who I am today. Thank you. My family, God, I love you guys so much—and that includes you, Andraia, and all the Bertinellis—just love. I can't say anything more or better. Just love. And the same to my girlfriends, who keep me grounded and happy. Ed, I love you and miss you. And Wolfie, my sweet, sweet boy—I love you to the moon and back. I am one ridiculously proud mama.

And a final message to the rest of the world: Enough already with anything that doesn't come from love. When we all make decisions based on love, we will be better and kinder.

# Recipe Index